WE
DON'T
USE
WORDS
LIKE
'CRAZY'

WE DON'T USE WORDS LIKE 'CRAZY'

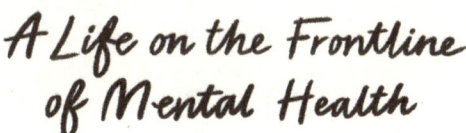

A Life on the Frontline of Mental Health

ELLIOT SWEENEY, RMN

First published in the UK in 2025 by Blink Publishing
An imprint of Bonnier Books UK
5th Floor, HYLO, 105 Bunhill Row,
London, EC1Y 8LZ

Copyright © Elliot Sweeney, 2025

All rights reserved.

No part of this publication may be reproduced, stored or transmitted in any form or by any means, electronic, mechanical, photocopying or otherwise, without the prior written permission of the publisher.

The right of Elliot Sweeney to be identified as Author of this work has been asserted by him in accordance with the Copyright, Designs and Patents Act, 1988.

A CIP catalogue record for this book is available from the British Library.

Hardback ISBN: 9781785122064

Also available as an ebook and an audiobook

1 3 5 7 9 10 8 6 4 2

Design and Typeset by Envy Design Ltd
Printed and bound in Great Britain by Clays Ltd, Elcograf S.p.A.

Every reasonable effort has been made to trace copyright holders of material reproduced in this book, but if any have been inadvertently overlooked the publishers would be glad to hear from them.

This book is a work of Non-Fiction. Some names have been changed to respect the privacy of those mentioned.

The authorised representative in the EEA is
Bonnier Books UK (Ireland) Limited.
Registered office address: Floor 3, Block 3, Miesian Plaza,
Dublin 2, D02 Y754, Ireland
compliance@bonnierbooks.ie

www.bonnierbooks.co.uk

For Spencer

This book contains material that may trigger emotional distress or discomfort for some readers, including discussion of self-harm and suicidal ideation.

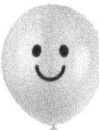

Contents

Foreword	ix
The Boy With the Thorn In His Side	1
Heaven Knows I'm Miserable Now	7
Every Day is Like Sunday	25
Still Ill	61
Maladjusted	93
Cemetery Gates	119
Sweet and Tender Hooligan	135
Girl Afraid	157
That Joke Isn't Funny Anymore	183
Suffer the Children	201
Some Girls are Bigger than Others	227
Stretch Out and Wait	245
There is a Light That Never Goes Out	271
Acknowledgements	275

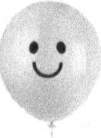

Foreword

THE AIM OF THIS book is to show what it's like working in contemporary mental health care. It's about the one in ten whose lives are affected by these kinds of illnesses; about those, like me, who make helping them their vocation; and about how, when you get down to brass tacks, the lines that separate these two groups are closer than they appear.

I want to share the bafflement and frustration, the boredom, shock, anger and laughter that comes on my beat; to journey onto understaffed wards, where industrial bleach and reheated dinner smells are seared by howls and alarms for response teams; I want you to hear first-hand of the loneliness the mentally ill experience, living in quiet desperation, being laughed at, stigmatised, forgotten; I want you to meet the mentally disordered offenders feared by society, nihilistic teenagers on the cusp of life, dementia patients approaching the end, and see how suffering speaks a universal language; I want you to feel the burnout, the compassion fatigue, the vicarious trauma those who work in this sector take home, and to hear about the raw hope, the quiet victories, and catch glimpses into the marrow of the human soul that keeps us going.

I want you to be shocked. I want you to be appalled, amused, provoked. I want you to ask difficult questions about your part in these problems, and how care of the mentally ill reflects the society in which we live.

Perhaps mental illness has affected you, or someone close to you. Perhaps you work in the field and are reading this for comparative reasons. Or perhaps, wrongly, you believe you know nothing.

Whatever, you are welcome. Be reassured that immense care has gone into upholding the real-life confidentiality of the people in this book. To this end, I've merged identities, amalgamated stories, changed individuals' genders and characteristics, added significant poetic licence, all to preserve patient anonymity without losing the pathos these stories carry. Any obvious similarities with actual people are coincidental.

Yet everything you are about to read is true.

The Boy With the Thorn In His Side

JACK, EIGHTEEN, HAS some good news.

'I'm ending your detention,' his consultant psychiatrist says. 'You've been in hospital three months. It's time to start thinking about the future.'

We are, Jack, the psychiatrist, Jack's mum, Mary, and me, a nurse trainee, in a stuffy office situated within the mental health ward Jack has been confined to.

Jack glances up, looks at his psychiatrist through his floppy mop top, and at me. Mary leans over, touches her son's hand that clasps his knee. His knuckles are white, the skin welted with dints and scars.

This is big news: it means Jack's no longer 'sectioned'. Now, he's an 'informal' patient, allowed to leave this ward and the hospital site of his own volition, and unaccompanied.

'See this as a positive,' the psychiatrist continues. 'All being well, you'll be home by the end of the week. Well done.' He glances at the wall clock: there's a crammed schedule of patients to get through, and we've already overshot. 'Well, better move on. Do you have any questions?'

Jack, the introverted, unusually sweet-mannered son of teachers, shrugs a signature shrug and says nothing. But is that the curvature of a smile I see?

'This *is* a positive,' I later tell him.

We're in his porridge-grey room furnished only with a few photos of Jack with his parents taped above the single bed (Blu-Tack is a no-no in the hospital after a patient ingested a large globule, and pins are an outright ban). Outside, the sounds of the ward pulse – a dry cackling cough; a droning TV shopping channel; a charge nurse announcing dinner time; a cry.

I'm leaning on the windowsill, looking at Jack; he's perched on the mattress, concentrating on his feet. Were it not for the NHS lanyard around my neck, it would look like two mates hanging out.

'It means the psychiatrist thinks you're ready for discharge,' I add.

'Right,' Jack says.

'So, what would you like to do when you get out?'

His lips tighten; he shakes his head. 'Don't know.'

'Uni?'

Shrug.

'Travel?'

Shrug.

'What about music? You wanted to get back into playing guitar, didn't you?'

'Right.'

'Maybe get a new one and start playing?'

'Maybe.'

'You've got to do something, mate. Not just wallow.'

With Jack, I can talk in this manner. We're a similar age, from a similar part of the city, with similar tastes, and I've spent a lot of time with him – one of the perks to being a trainee not yet bogged down with admin and medication checks like the qualified nurses. We've grown close, Jack and me. I know him.

This admission came off the back of an overdose of paracetamol, triggered by a relapse in Jack's bipolar-affective disorder. Compared to how he was when he was first admitted, he's made strides – washing, shaving, accepting his lithium despite the side-effects, talking, albeit grudgingly, about his mental health, reclaiming a semblance of who he was.

We've spent hours together, waxing over the best Nirvana album (*In Utero*, of course); who was the master wordsmith, Hemingway or Fitzgerald (prior to the breakdown, Jack had been poised to start a literature degree); I've administered his meds, supervised his meals, escorted his leave, even delivered a rapid tranquiliser into his gluteal muscle when he became particularly agitated. We've been through a lot together. I'm happy for him.

'You better start planning, then,' I say.

'Right,' Jack says.

'I'm expecting to hear about your band topping the charts this time next year.'

'Right.'

'Fist pump?'

We touch skin.

A day later, Jack takes advantage of his newfound freedom.

WE DON'T USE WORDS LIKE 'CRAZY'

It's one of those summer mornings in London, the air balmy, thick with a polluted, savage kind of heat.

After breakfast, he leaves the hospital alone and takes a shaded half-mile stroll down a hill to the nearest parade of shops and a tube station. The support workers who see him later remark that he seems quite himself as he passes and says 'hi'. Nothing untoward.

The next turn of events is less clear. I know from the police report that he buys two bottles of fizzy drink and a guitar magazine from a convenience store before entering the tube station. Shopping bags in hand, he taps through the gate, descends the escalator, walks to the southbound platform, takes a seat on a bench. CCTV shows him drink both bottles and leaf through the magazine for ten minutes.

Then, as the eyes of a train light the tunnel, he walks to the platform edge and climbs onto the tracks.

I find out the next morning. It's the start of shift; handover in the nursing station. The scene is crystalised in my memory. 'I Don't Feel Like Dancin'' by Scissor Sisters prattles from the radio. Instant coffee smells swirl in the static air.

And Jack is dead.

I place my tea on the desk, ask the shift lead, a stucco-chinned charge nurse, what he's talking about.

'He's dead,' he repeats. 'Hadn't you heard?'

No, I hadn't heard.

I ask for details. Get told them.

The words swim.

It reaches the local press. A young man granted leave from a secure mental hospital kills himself by leaping under a rush-hour train. It seems so avoidable. But it doesn't cause the furore I expect, perhaps hope for. When I ask colleagues why, they roll eyes, shrug, smile wryly, and explain:

Jack was a mental health patient.

Mental health patients do crazy things.

It's what people expect.

Isn't it?

A week later, as is Trust policy, those of us who knew Jack are invited to a staff debrief. In a poky conference room, where an ancient photocopier and overhead projectors have been bundled into a corner gathering dust, we sit in a circle and are encouraged to reflect.

One by one, colleagues speak. Someone comments that suicide is a part of the job; someone else calls it an 'occupational hazard'. There are murmurs of agreement. Above our heads, the strip-lighting flickers.

I sit, one leg over the other, arms folded tight. There's so much noise in my head, things I want to throw out. Was Jack's death impulsive? Or was he planning it in advance? If it was planned, why buy the fizzy drinks and magazine? And why the hell hadn't he told me?

'Elliot,' someone says, 'do you want to share something?'

I shake my head.

At the inquest, six months later, we're told that Jack had serious mental health problems, and no faults are cited in the care and support he received on the ward.

A few of my colleagues from the ward, Jack's schoolfriends, his muted parents and me, now a newly qualified mental health nurse, hear the coroner explain how he'd shown positive signs of recovery in the days prior to his death. This was why his detention was ended, and he'd been allowed to leave the ward. Jack's death was tragic. But in mental health, tragedies happen.

This should cut it. Death is part of the job. Toughen up, I tell myself.

By now, I've studied textbooks, watched documentaries and films on the causes and effects of psychiatric disorders like the one Jack had. On paper, the act of self-destruction has always held a dark romantic interest, with Ian Curtis, Kurt Cobain and Richey Manic three well-known suicides I'm familiar with. Their abrupt ends seem to somehow elevate their craft, proving they were indisputably the 'real deal', eulogising their stories, turning '. . . disaster into art', as Al Alvarez poignantly wrote of his friend Sylvia Plath's death.

But Jack's suicide is different. He isn't leaving a legacy, a body of posthumous work to plough through. No, Jack was an awkward young man. He'd died a sad, violent death, driven by something in him, a malignancy of his mind. There were no blood tests for it, no clear consensus of what defined it. But it made the prospect of living unbearable.

As I watch Jack's parents leave the coroner's court, leaning into one another, eyes flat and dead in contrast with the bloom of spring, it all hits me, and a void seems to stretch out beyond the confines of my skull.

How do I feel?

Right then, I feel cold, harsh, shitty, and very, very young.

Heaven Knows
I'm Miserable Now

JACK'S DEATH STILL feels cold, harsh and shitty. But I've stuck at this job and been weathered by others since.

Whenever I supervise someone new to this unusual sector, I try to emphasise the perks of the job – the breadth of individuals you'll meet, the positive interventions you can make, the remarkable backstories you'll hear. But I also stress that it isn't a case of *if* but *when* a patient they care for will complete (not commit, never, ever 'succeed' in) a suicide.

Paediatrics, oncology, emergency medicine – death is a reality in any health setting: the 'occupational hazard', as my crass but insightful colleague had said. But suicide feels like a different animal, doesn't it? Rather than the closing answer to illness or pain, taking one's life – abruptly, alone and in acute crisis – is steeped in uncomfortable questions. And invariably, they remain unanswered. Jack's death altered me. I became aware that mental health is a serious business: illnesses of the mind are as fatal as heart attacks.

In normal life, describing what goes on in mental health services provokes looks of horror. And recounting stories like Jack's is always a great way to kill a party. But when you work in this peculiar sector of health care they are bread and butter, mulled over with a brew in the office. Topics I've discussed this week include autoerotic asphyxiation, bleach drinking, cutlery swallowing, auto-amputation, coprophilia, necrophilia, defenestration, emasculation and self-emollition as a practicable means of suicide. And it's only Thursday.

Surviving this work demands a stoic sheet of armour, a doggedness around life's hardships and inequities, and a pretty dark sense of humour to boot.

Over the years, I've come up with theories for why Jack did what he did. The medication he was prescribed would have had grisly side-effects: weight gain; raised blood pressure; excessive salivation; flatness of mood; fluid retention; erectile dysfunction; facial hair (in both men and women) and milk lactation (in both men and women). Grim stuff for anyone to tolerate, especially so if you're a young adult on the cusp of life.

There's the damage to the fledgling sense of identity he would have felt too, being tarred with the mental health brush. The otherness. The anger. The dismay. He'd have known that he had an affliction – chronic, pernicious, misunderstood; it would make his future uncertain, affect his travel plans, driving, relationships. His friends, peers, lovers, future employers would look at him differently. Because he *was* different.

I'd like to think that Jack experienced moments of genuine hope while I knew him, flashes of confidence I saw that were real to him. But mental illnesses are master infiltrators – they know all the tricks you do, and work as hard as you to claw you back down.

Ultimately, we'll never know what he was thinking when he took that walk to the train station, read his magazine, drank his pop and made his final gesture. We only know the outcome.

Herein lies a harsh uniquity of mental health care – we can never say how many lives we've saved; we only know for certain those we've lost.

Be honest, if someone you know got diagnosed with a major mental disorder and sent to hospital in the way Jack was, what thoughts would come to mind?

Before I embarked on this career, I can tell you where my head would've gone – to the movies. Anthony Hopkins in *The Silence of the Lambs* as Hannibal Lecter, the cannibalistic psychopath strapped to the gurney, a hockey mask encaging smirking red lips stretched wide around small white teeth. Russell Crowe in *A Beautiful Mind* as maths genius and paranoid schizophrenic John Nash, waxing with a best friend and little girl for half the film before he and the audience realise these are hallucinations no one else can see. Béatrice Dalle in sultry erotic French tragedy *Betty Blue*, delivering a raw, rampant depiction of personality disorder in the barest flesh – hysteric, punching mirrors, gouging out her eye before getting strapped to a bed and medicated to her (remaining) eyeball.

Perhaps the biggest imprint was left by Miloš Forman's *One Flew Over the Cuckoo's Nest*. Released in 1975, and based upon Ken Kesey's allegorical, counterculture novel, this Oscar winner is set within Oregon State Hospital. The sweetly sadistic Nurse Ratched and her staff of uniformed thugs maintain a veneer of order through multifaceted disempowerment of the patients, a scathing metaphor for the societal constraints Kesey's generation punched against.

I remember seeing the film on a rented VHS as a twelve-year-old: it had a profound effect. Jack Nicholson plays Randle McMurphy, a rambunctious criminal faking madness to swerve prison before realising his mistake. His defiance to Ratched's subjugation prompts his fellow patients to reclaim agency over their lives, but it seals his own fate in the process.

At one point, McMurphy receives electroconvulsive therapy (ECT), used punitively and without anaesthetic. This infamous scene, which patients still ask about, is horrifically executed, the electric shock inducing a violent seizure, coiling McMurphy's spine into an arc and forcing veins to web the surface of his beetroot skin. Thankfully, the depiction is wholly inaccurate. But the impression was left on me.

Work by celebs with lived experience – Frank Bruno, Gail Porter and Stephen Fry to name a few – and charities such as *MIND* and *Rethink* have helped demystify these skewed Hollywood depictions, showing that mental health issues are commonplace, and treatments humane; drives like World Mental Health Day and the Campaign Against Living Miserably (CALM) have furthered the cause, raising the agenda, getting us talking, opening up, being real.

Despite all this, the preconceptions, presumptions and

outright prejudices breathe on. Mentally ill people are dangerous. Mental health hospitals are like prisons. You'd have to be crazy to work in one of those places.

Wouldn't you?

'So, you want to be a registered *male* nurse?'

'No, Margaret.' I glance at my girlfriend Clare, presently hiding her laugh behind a mug of tea. 'RMN stands for registered *mental health* nurse. Being male has nothing to do with it.'

Margaret, Clare's grandmother, gives a confused stare.

We, Clare and I, are visiting her in her flat in Nelson, a small grey town in east Lancashire. After telling her about our journey up from London, holiday plans, and hearing Margaret reminisce about Clare as a girl, I decided to tell her my career plan.

'What will you do then?' Margaret says. 'As a *mental health* nurse?'

'I'll help people,' I say. 'You know, with difficult thoughts and emotions.'

'How's that done?'

I shrug. 'Through talking and stuff.'

'Stuff?'

I nod. *Yeah. Stuff.*

In a couple of weeks, I'll start a diploma in mental health nursing, training at a former polytechnic in a dusty suburb of northwest London; it's a two-year course leading to a professional registration with the Nursing and Midwifery Council.

'You give medicines though, don't you?' Margaret asks. 'Like proper nurses?'

'Mental health nurses *are* proper nurses, Margaret,' I say, smiling. 'It's just a different speciality. But there's more to it than pills. There's building relationships. Earning trust. Standing shoulder to shoulder with people while they're going through a rubbish time.'

'What if they stab you?'

The smile crumbles.

'That's unlikely, Gran,' Clare says.

'The mentally ill are more risk to themselves than others,' I add.

The confused stare returns. 'Well, I don't understand. In my day, people just got on with things. What will you do? Day to day, I mean?'

I hesitate.

It was a hard question then, and it remains so. Roles I've performed as a mental health nurse include: hair washer, pill popper, bum wiper, injection giver, punch dodger, hand holder, inquest attender; I've been a custodian, comedian, confidante, carpenter, colleague, advocate and friend.

Some mental health nurses consider themselves hard-science clinicians, with brain scans and blood tests, psychiatric jargon and medical pathology their discourse; others liken themselves to therapeutic, holistic, even artistic practitioners, seeing the nurse as a companion to those in acute distress; a few draw comparisons with the prison officer, versed in restraining and monitoring, there to maintain order, compliance, oversight; and a small number are perhaps drawn to this field because it placates, even treats, their own mental health issues.

Opinions about what defines the mental health nurse split during the 1960s and '70s, a dynamic time in psychiatry.

Before then, care of the mentally ill was a belt and braces medical discipline, and the aetiology and treatment of these illnesses was largely medicalised. A growing momentum of critics pushed against this approach, with psychiatrist R.D. Laing in the UK, philosopher Michel Foucault in France, and the infamous Thomas Szasz in the States all offering compelling social narratives and biting critiques.

Szasz said, 'Most people we call mentally ill impersonate the role of helpless, hopeless, when, in fact, their actual roles pertain to frustration, unhappiness and perplexities.'

These *anti*-psychiatry voices asked people to consider that the problems didn't lie with the mentally ill but with us, a society unwilling to tolerate difference and peculiarity.

So where did I fit into all this? In answer to Margaret's question, what would I do, day to day?

'I don't really know,' I say, truthfully. 'But I'm looking forward to finding out.'

'Well,' she says, 'congratulations on your career choice. If it makes you happy. Rather you than me though.' She reaches for the custard creams, then pauses. 'But what made you want to do a job like this in the first place?'

There is a heavy pause.

'I need the loo,' I say, and scurry to the kitchen, leaving the silence in the room swinging like a body on a noose.

Questions I've been asked about being a mental health nurse:

'Gosh, doesn't that drive you a bit mental too?'

'I mean, don't you find it kind of harrowing?'

'Man, I bet you've seen some fucked-up shit?'

To all these, I can answer a resolute yes, make a dark joke, maybe tell a story or two, or go quiet. Margaret's question is the most common though, and perhaps the hardest to answer: 'What made you want to do a job like this?'

I suspect the idea was germinating in the compost of my mind for a while, but the first time I became aware of it was during the spring of 1998 . . .

The internet is a new phenomenon. New Labour have been in government for a year. *TFI Friday* hogs the telly, Britpop the airwaves, Man United the league. We drink Hooch and Smirnoff Ice, read *Loaded* and *FHM*, wear 8-hole DMs, Adidas track-tops and smoke Marlboro Lights in pubs with impunity. Some book about a boy wizard is starting a furore, and if you'd mentioned Brexit or Covid, you might think they were characters in that same wizarding book.

Situated on a leafy elbow of London is my school, the largest comp in the borough. It's a sprawling mishmash of turn-of-the-century red brick and drab 1970s prefabs with a sixth form soldered on. My memory is of mustard-yellow cladding and bin-liner brown filing cabinets, fluorescent strip lights, marker pens squeaking on white boards, and hordes of angsty kids, like me.

I'm seventeen, mercurial, guitar wielding, Oasis obsessed. I'm craving experience, painfully *un*aware of how much there is to learn, but dangerously certain I know it all. Everything blasts in technicolour – hopes, ambitions, desires. It's a vibrant, visceral time.

Amid these memories, there's a bowl-cut piano prodigy from my music class. His name is Terry. Terry has a mental illness. But no one knows that yet.

He's eccentric, with his loquacious manner, disregard for fashion and slang. There's his piercing brown eyes, Fair Isle jumpers, moccasin shoes; his wild jazz improvs, large, flapping hands, his slightly crazy laugh. Terry's a polymath; as well as music, he can do maths, writing, philosophy, drinking and, I'll later learn, smoking large quantities of cannabis. Even though he's loud and garrulous, with a tendency to invade personal space and shoot spittle when he talks, he's popular – a warm, kooky kid. Everyone knows he's going places.

Unsurprisingly, Terry smashes his A-levels, top marks all the way. I, on the other hand, get Bs and Cs, my daydreaming and dyslexia holding me back.

That summer, Terry heads off to Oxbridge to read PPE (Philosophy, Politics and Economics). Meanwhile, my band, who I'd firmly believed were destined for stardom, implodes. In grief, I take up work at a rock'n'roll pub in Camden, discover E, illegal raves, Raymond Chandler, the opposite sex. I get my heart broken, nearly my nose too, and the first of many stupid tattoos.

The best part of a year goes by. LeAnn Rimes fights the Spice Girls for the number-one spot. The IRA bomb Omagh, the worst terrorist atrocity in the UK to date. Ted Hughes, husband of the late Sylvia Plath, dies.

I next see Terry at the pub. It's football derby day, Arsenal versus Spurs. The place is packed, lads from when we were at school sporting footie tops, goatee beards, clutching pints of Stella like badges of pride. It's a raucous place, reeking of Lynx, fags, hops and testosterone.

I spot Terry sitting at a small table, a drink, deck of Lights and an overflowing ashtray his companions. He isn't watching the wall-mounted screen showing the game. He's focused entirely on his pint, the bubbles rising to the surface.

At half-time, Des Lynam and big Ron Atkinson begin their critiques, and I head over. Close up, Terry's skin is puffy. The moccasins have holes and his jumper and jeans are stained and scuffed; his bowl-cut is matted, peppered with dandruff; he's put on weight, with stubbly jowls, his neck doughy; a loose tyre hangs over the hem of his jeans.

But that's not all. Terry's expression, his demeanour, have altered. Lips curved downwards. Eyes half-mast. A sense of profound inwardness. Later, I will learn about negative symptoms of mental disorder, those that rob the sufferer of facets of their former self, leaving them like a marionette with its strings snipped. But right then, all I know is something is lacking in my old schoolfriend.

'Terry.'

His eyes find mine. Recognition shines dimly through the mist.

'El.' His teeth are bad, a tea-stained colour; even from a distance I can smell his musty, smoky breath. We shake hands. Sweaty palms, limp grip, long, dirty fingernails.

'Good to see you, mate,' I say.

He nods.

'Enjoying uni?'

'I dropped out.'

I wait for more. Nothing.

'Why'd you do that?' I say.

'A few problems.'

'Oh, sorry, man. Is everything OK?' I hesitate. 'Are you OK?'

He nods again, says, 'I'm calm.'

Calm. An odd thing to say, not really an answer, but perhaps meant as a good thing. After all, the Terry I remembered always was a little woo-woo.

'I'm on meds,' he adds.

I clear my throat. Right, he's sick. Up till now, I've never had a friend who's ill before, but I'm a grown-up. I can handle this. I want to pry, to ask what his ailment is. But something keeps the questions at bay. Instead, we sit opposite each other, not speaking.

'I'm getting more fags,' he eventually says, and heads for the machine.

I stay where I am, trying to think of something to say next. I'm still trying when it dawns on me that he's not coming back. While I'd been thinking, Terry pushed through the swinging double doors into the harsh daylight.

Later, a mate mooches over, someone else from our school. 'Saw you talking to Terry,' he says, a little slurry.

I nod.

'He say anything mental?'

'Not really,' I say. 'Why?'

He throws an arm around my shoulder, shouts into my ear, 'Guess you haven't heard?'

'Heard what?'

'Terry's got *schiz-o-fre-nee-a*.' Each syllable is enunciated slowly, as if he's talking to a child.

I ask him to repeat what he'd said. He repeats it, even louder. I hadn't misheard. Then he laughs and heads to the bar, inviting me to go with him. I stay put.

Schizophrenia.

Schizo.
Psycho.
The pub suddenly seems to empty.
I'm confused. Scared too. And I don't know why.

It turned out that while at university, Terry's cannabis use graduated to LSD and ketamine, along with pub crawls, sleep deprivation and academic stress. He began missing lectures and assignment deadlines, avoiding newfound friends and mates from back home; he sent rambling emails to tutors and family, stating his intentions to abandon his studies and become a preacher, as he'd found the mystery to life when God spoke to him in a dream.

His parents grew concerned and contacted the student support services, who, it transpired, already had Terry on their radar. A psychiatrist was asked to visit his halls room, found Terry naked in bed wearing a large beard, thin and wan, muttering to spirits only he could see. An admission to a local hospital was promptly arranged, where he was sectioned under the Mental Health Act to prevent him leaving.

What everyone hoped would be a brief stay turned into three months on a locked ward, during which time Terry's quasi-existential beliefs became more obscure. He saw patterns in books, heard messages on TV programmes, all telling him he was a deity at the centre of an existential puzzle and he had to leave the UK immediately to save mankind.

He was commenced on a course of antipsychotics, switched to another when they had little impact, and eventually, these beliefs – tagged as delusions of grandeur – began to temper;

it was around this time he was also given a diagnosis of paranoid schizophrenia.

Some of this I gleaned from friends, other bits from Terry himself. For I continued to bump into him over the years that followed, normally spotting him on a stool beneath the awning of a coffee shop, smoking, staring searchingly. In that time, his appearance continued to change. His hair greyed and receded and his skin turned flaccid, like a deflated balloon. His fingernails grew long and nicotine yellow and his eyes bore a strained, haunted look. He was still Terry, but a blunted version. Some of this was caused by the antipsychotic meds, I'm sure of this now; but the rest came from his illness itself, not to mention the crushing impact living with a label like schizophrenia must have.

I can remember bumping into him on one occasion outside a Costa. Terry wears a grubby charity shop coat, tracksuit bottoms and slippers. He stares at me flatly. A shrewd, sharp mind is now an unctuous glue. I ask how he is.

'The jigsaw's been put back together,' he says. 'But some of the pieces of the puzzle are in the wrong place. And I can't figure out how to fix them.'

An elegant metaphor, a glimpse that the Terry I remember is still there somewhere. But proof that there's something irretrievable in him too.

'I'm sorry, mate,' is all I can think to say.

A short time later, I feel ready for a new vocation. I hang up my barman's towel and sign up with a social care agency covering London and the southeast. When the agency asks me what kind of work I'd like to do, I immediately express an interest in mental health care. If you'd asked me why, I'd have told you it was because the agency paid seventy pence more an hour to support this unpopular client group.

But that's not the real reason.

A match had been struck. I'm ready to see more.

Within days, I have a job at a residential home for adults living with 'enduring mental health issues'. Whatever that means.

This home has the look of a Dickensian workhouse, cramped and grubby, Terracotta walls and pus-grey masonry, the interior reeking of damp, fags and mould. It's incongruously located between Covent Garden and Holborn – prime London real estate, an old Peabody building adjacent to a well-known gents' clothing retailer from where razor-jeaned fashionistas stare out with befuddled fear at the residents coming and going.

These residents (also called service users, customers, beneficiaries, ad infinitum) are the offcuts from those vast mental asylums built during the last century, many closed during the era of 'care in the community' in the early 1990s. They are folk from all walks, unified by their illnesses, and institutionalised from years spent away. We have daughters of aristocrats, down and outs scooped off the Strand, a former sergeant-major, even a one-time vicar; but most have never worked or lived independently, or ever will – I soon recognise the Largactil shuffle, the dyskinesia twitches, the dysphonic slur, the Parkinsonian retardations that first-generation antipsychotics have left them with. My job is to support them to live the lives they want to live while protecting them from harm. Simple.

HEAVEN KNOWS I'M MISERABLE NOW

To this end, I dish out meds, slap up wallpaper, tend dry feet, deliver pressure sore care, cut hair, shave beards, receive abuse – and one or two compliments. I feed, water, wash, dry, accompany to the offie, the cinema, Buckingham Palace and Soho sex shops. I laugh with some residents over half a pint and a game of darts, share cigarettes, stick up for them when people stare and cajole, cry with them when one of them is found dead.

It's hard work, hands-on, gritty and not a million miles away from working in the pub. I go home smelling of smoke and must, my shoes sticky from walking in tobacco-strewn, syrup-encrusted floors. But compared to the jobs my mates from school have started, working in offices, banks, car showrooms, advertising firms, this feels decidedly real.

The thirty-one residents in the home exist in a ramshackle community as rich and diverse as any in the city. When I listen past their peculiarities, their word-salad dialects, I hear extraordinary tales: surviving conversion therapy to 'cure' homosexuality; undergoing rebirthing and exorcisms to rid demons; attending Kingsley Hall in the 1960s, where staff and patients coexisted with equanimity, holding hands, chanting, being rebirthed; sharing a ward, and a bed, with Syd Barrett from Pink Floyd, whose fingernails curled like undulating rollercoaster tracks. They are remarkable, hilarious, sometimes awful stories a writer would pull his teeth for. It doesn't take long for me to fall for mental health work, and to see myself making a career of it.

Every few weeks, a psychiatrist visits to check up on the residents. He's a likeable if insouciant chap with an alphabet of letters after his name; he dresses in expensive suits, speaks with an expensive accent, asks if there are any 'issues', rhyming the first syllable with 'piss'. He tweaks medication doses, asks about side-effects, almost making eye contact as he scribes notes with a Parker fountain pen.

I watch, considering his role. Clearly, the man knows a huge amount about mental illness. Upon Googling his name, I find reams of publications he's penned – longitudinal trials, double-bind experiments, medication studies. But he isn't talking to the residents the way I would want to be spoken to. There's a distance, a detachment.

Seeing myself as a psychiatrist seems far-fetched. I have neither the academic grades nor the inclination to attempt six years of med school, train to be a doctor and follow this career path.

But some of the mental health nurses joining him on his rounds spark my interest. These guys wear DMs, have bad tats and piercings; they smoke, drink, like music and football, and, best of all, they talk to the residents – *really* talk to them.

Alan, a jocular nurse from Glasgow, makes an impression. We get on. Outside the care home one afternoon, while he's making a roll-up, I mention I'm thinking of training to be a nurse.

After croaking out his twenty-a-day laugh, he says, 'You're not serious?'

I tell him I am.

'Well, it's a tough job.'

'I know.'

'Why do you want to do it?'

'I don't know,' I say. 'Why do you do it?'

'Not for the money. Definitely not for the thanks I get.' He licks the gum of his Rizla paper, puts the cigarette to his mouth.

I try to think of something to ask. While I do, he sparks up, and through a cloud he gives me one of the best bits of advice I've had: 'Spend a morning on a busy acute ward. I'll arrange it for you, if you like. That'll put you off.'

I fall silent.

An acute mental health ward. The epicentre of frontline mental health care. The sort of place where they locked up Terry. Until now, I've never set foot on one.

Images of straitjackets, padded cells and men in white coats flood my mind. This is where the florid psychotics, the catatonic depressives, the self-harmers, haters and bona fide loonies get lumbered.

'Well?' Alan says.

I say nothing.

'You scared?'

'No,' I lie.

He chuckles, and suddenly he seems distant; I feel myself suspended in the wide expanse. My lips tingle, and my fingertips go numb; I've slipped into a fugue, yet I'm intensely aware of my surroundings, the gum-coated pavement, the smoky air.

'Well, think about it,' Alan says. 'Let me know if–'

'I'll do it,' I blurt.

His eyebrows rise. 'Then I'll make a call,' he says, adding, 'Don't worry. You'll be fine.'

And I have been fine. Mostly.

That first visit to a mental health ward, arranged by Alan, took me to a central London hospital near Pimlico. Immediately after that I filled out an application to study mental health nursing. It was a done deal.

My mates scoffed when I told them, or they looked at me warily. I was always creative at school, telling people I'd grow up to make music or write books. They asked the same question Clare's grandmother asked: why would I want to be a mental health nurse?

Why wouldn't I? Already I knew the authenticity found in mental health care is without comparison. There's no pretence or posturing. You see people raw, stripped of trappings, exposed, without fluffy filters. Painfully human. Experiencing human pain like no other.

But describing it is one thing, being there is quite different.

In the next chapter, I'd like you to do as I did. That's right: you're going to step foot onto a modern-day mental health ward much like the one I first did, meet the same staff and patients I recall from that first visit, and be there. I want you to ask questions, breathe in the same air. I want you to listen.

Scared? I was too.

Don't worry. You'll be fine.

Every Day is Like Sunday

THE LUNATICS ACT of the mid-nineteenth century placed a statutory requirement on local authorities to provide secure environments for the mad and feeble-minded. Traditionally, these were asylums, holding pens for society's undesirables, with Bethlem – aka Bedlam – being the most renowned, and notorious.

These establishments are now called mental health hospitals, facilities, units or suchlike. They are as complex and diverse as the people they serve, but the overarching aim is simple: the care and treatment of those suffering disorders of the mind.

The mental health hospital will often be christened with a picturesque title – The Beach, The Farmyard, The Stables, you get the idea, to divert us from its function and the grim connotations. They are dotted around the country, excrescences you may have seen in passing but then pushed aside in your mind. Oddities and eyesores, intriguing yet repellent, akin to lifejackets on a cruise ship – you're glad they're there, but God forbid you ever need to make use of them.

Some mental health hospitals are aged, gothic structures, prone to leaks, subsidence and all manner of decline; some are modern, purpose-built, looming complexes, characterless, utilitarian, harsh; some are attached onto pre-existing general hospital sites, the barred windows and amalgamation of smokers outside the giveaway about the clientele.

However the exterior appears, within these mental health hospitals there will be various mental health wards. Some care for patients with specific conditions: there are eating disorder wards, mother and baby wards, older adult wards, child and adolescent wards, male-only wards, female-only wards, psychiatric intensive care units (PICU); there are outpatient wards, day unit wards, crisis wards.

But mostly, wards are mixed acute, containing men and women from eighteen to sixty-five, all presenting with some kind of serious mental illness that warrants them being there.

These are dynamic places, with high turnarounds of patients and staff. Yet in the same way that charity shops all smell of mothballs, mental health wards share ubiquitous traits.

You're going to visit one such ward. It holds up to thirty patients. And like all mental health wards in the UK, it's always, always full.

Let's get the bed crisis issue out of the way now. The dearth of mental health hospital capacity has reached epidemic proportions during the last decade, the worst I've ever known it. Patients are waiting days, sometimes weeks for a bed they urgently need, during which time they remain in a community setting, deteriorating, sometimes dying avoidable deaths. Meantime, discharges of patients are being hampered due to the crumbling social care system and cuts to charity and universal aid. It means some patients are staying in beds they don't need, blocking essential throughput.

In desperation, NHS trusts are put under increasing pressure to facilitate premature discharges, either sending sick patients home, to hotels and B&Bs, or to private hospitals. That's right, I'm talking about those fluffy places you read about in the noughties where celebs used to go to dry out – they are now all havens for acute mental health patients, costing thousands of taxpayers' pounds, all because there's not enough beds in the NHS anymore. Madness.

Your ward is within an old-fashioned NHS mental hospital of the standard Victorian type. The exterior is red brick and grey limestone, a linear model with wings radiating off the main block so that all the corridors have an unobstructed view. This is a penal architecture, pragmatic, engrained with regularity, organisation and flagrant disregard for style.

The only vibrancy comes from the perimeter walls. A fluttering of flowers and shrubs is bedded in wooden barrels beneath the THANK YOU FOR NOT SMOKING sign by the main entrance. A portly man in a dressing gown and slippers stands beneath the sign, tugging on a roll-up, flicking ash into the azaleas. He eyes you as you pass him and step through double doors into the main reception, a narrow rectangular space with more doors on either side.

Ahead, an administrator is ensconced behind opaque glass, typing on her keyboard. Above her, taped to the wall is the word WELC ME, the O appearing to have fallen off. Listless piano keys tinkle from a Roberts Radio on a sill.

Next to this there's a table of donated books, a hot drinks dispenser, a large TV showing a muted daytime quiz.

You approach, tap the glass, make eye contact with the administrator, smile. Her flowery dress jars with her steely expression. You explain why you're here. She stops typing, checks her logbook. The piano music tinkles.

'Through you go,' she says, indicating towards the door to the right. 'Follow the signs.'

'Shouldn't someone come with me?' you say.

She looks at you as if you'd just asked for a knife and fork at McDonald's, and then presses a button. On cue, an electromagnetic lock on the door makes a deep *wha-dum*. You push through, step into a corridor. Floors are shiny laminate, walls lime green. The air is warm and bleachy.

The door thuds shut behind you, another heavy *wha-dum*. Now you're locked in. You take in this artery that will lead into the heart of the hospital, and the piano music outside, still audible, slips into a minor key.

You follow signs towards the wards, passing doors that say pharmacy, chaplaincy, tribunal room, ECT suite. The bleachy smell grows tart, and you realise it's masking the clag of stale bodies. As you curve inwards, your attention is caught by paintings framed on the wall – patient artwork, you realise, encased behind thick Perspex.

You're taking in a picture of a pedal boat on a lake when a different door *wha-dum*s ahead. Two figures emerge, both men. One is tall and bald, one short and bald. The tall one is dressed for the office, grey slacks, starched shirt, Windsor tie, salesman's smile. The short one is bedraggled. Ripped jeans, a motheaten jersey, a furtive stare.

Both stare at you.

'Morning,' the tall one says.

'Morning back,' you reply. 'Off out?'

'Escorted leave.' He indicates towards his companion, who mutters something incoherent.

Jargon buster: escorted leave describes a detained or 'sectioned' patient being allowed out with a staff member for a set period of time, perhaps to visit the supermarket, perhaps to meet with a friend or family member for a coffee, or just to go for some air and feel human.

Supporting patients out of the confines of the hospital and into the unpredictable outdoors is an unpopular job. Patients can push boundaries, refuse to leave shops, or to head back to their units. I've known some who've used leave to buy paracetamol, illicit drugs, razors, scissors, to run into traffic or take themselves to bridges.

But granting a patient leave should be maximised, helping avoid dependence or institutionalisation, returning a semblance of their basic human rights. When it works, it is empowering, but when it goes wrong, as it did with Jack, the results can be devastating.

This duo heads for the reception area, and you head for the ward they came from. The door is hefty, plated, and wouldn't look out of place on a submarine bough. CARING, NOT JUDGING, a sign reads. You press the buzzer, enthused by this sentiment.

Nothing happens.

You press again.

A yelp from behind the door, like a dog being trodden on.

Your finger is hovering over the buzzer once more when

there's the familiar magnetic *wha-dum*, and the door opens a few inches.

A slight, silver-haired man in a navy tunic and matching bottoms stands in the entranceway. His ID reveals his name to be Paul – a mental health nurse. He looks at you with sharp eyes, like a lip-reader's.

'Yes?' he says.

'Hello,' you say, and introduce yourself, explain why you're here. Your mouth is gummy dry as you speak.

'Come in, then,' Paul says, a little harried, and holds the door open enough for you to slip through. 'Welcome to the mad house,' he adds under his breath. Suddenly you are entering the ward, crossing a threshold most people will never have cause to do.

What were you expecting? Figures writhing on the floor? Gnashing teeth and straitjackets? Blood and faeces streaked up walls? In fact, you're on another characterless corridor. The walls are chipped, an off-grey colour slopped with clumsy cover-up paint strokes; the laminate flooring is bleary, reflecting the fluorescent strip lights overhead, the tubes scattered with crinkled fly corpses.

The tang of industrial bleach is cloying but cannot mask the reheated food smells, stale vape exhalations and meaty sweat. There's the clatter of pans from a kitchen, the rumble of a dryer, a beeping alarm. You can't see any patients yet; but you hear them, laughing, mewling, weeping.

'Hold tight,' Paul says behind you. 'Just sorting this out.'

You turn. And let out a gasp.

Directly to the right of the door is a thin woman at odds with the world. She's anywhere between thirty and sixty, wearing lime-green hospital bottoms that hang from her jutting hips like a bed sheet pinned to a drying frame. Her billowy T-shirt bears a smiley face saying: 'Have a Nice Day!' You realise where the yelp you heard earlier came from.

Her sinewy arms poke out the shirt, hands clawing, the fingers yellow. Her hair is grey, long, matted, framing the jagged oval of her gaunt face from which two pellet eyes watch you. There's dark suspicion in those eyes, and a secret, spiralling mirth – a mirth that echoes in the dark and seeps from cracks in the earth.

Presently, you know nothing about this woman. But you're sure of two things: she's a patient; and her mind is an unquiet place.

'Meet Emily,' Paul says. 'She's been trying to sneak out of here all morning, haven't you, Em?'

'Hi,' Emily says, in a surprisingly posh accent. She smiles a jagged smile, and it feels all wrong, with a coquettishness that tightens a knot in you.

'Hi,' you say back, your voice wobbly. Perhaps this could be an opportunity to build some rapport with a real-life patient, you think. 'Why do you want to leave? Don't you like it he–?'

Paul shakes his head.

Too late.

Emily starts screaming. It's a piercing keen that ricochets off the walls and ceiling like a bullet in a bank vault. You step back to a wall, hands out in feeble defence, feeling like a choirboy who's stumbled into an MMA cage.

'I don't belong here! Help! Help!'

You know the feeling.

'Easy, Em,' Paul says between her cries, manoeuvring himself slickly to her side, almost touching her shoulder, but not quite. 'Weren't you going to tell me about your grandson? How he's captain of the football team?'

Emily looks at Paul. Her mouth is agape. You're sure she's about to scream again.

But she doesn't. Instead, she stares up at Paul, who looks directly at her and says, 'Let's get you that cup of tea. You're safe here, my love.'

She inhales, exhales, her breath shuddering like she's on the back end of an asthma attack. Paul smiles, and then gently, skilfully, he begins ushering her away from the door, talking the whole time.

They call this redirecting: it's not rocket science, just a simple diverting technique, positively engaging the patient away from their focal point of stress towards something else, becoming their ally in the process.

You can't make out what Paul is saying as they walk off, but hearing the timbre of his voice is enough: a mix of warmth and assertion. In this moment you know that he's a skilled clinician, unfazed, and where a general nurse might use a canular or stethoscope, he's using words, his humanity, as tools.

Time passes. You remain against the wall. When Paul returns, you still haven't moved.

'Right then,' he says, smiling. 'Hope that hasn't scared you off already?' You try to say it hasn't, but it comes out something between a cough and a croak.

Paul chuckles.

'I'm sorry,' you stutter. 'Was that my fault?'

He shakes his head. 'Emily's a regular here. Keeps trying to escape. We can't let her do that. She's on a section.'

A section, sectioning, getting sectioned – all colloquialisms associated with the Mental Health Act, the legislative framework for mental illness in the UK. Knowing which patients are on a section, and which are not, is important for staff like Paul. Letting a sectioned patient off a ward can be catastrophic; likewise, refusing a voluntary patient to leave is an unlawful breach of their rights. Both can get you in serious trouble.

'Emily has a history of schizophrenia,' Paul continues. 'She's convinced we're conspiring against her.'

'She seems to like you.'

'For now,' he says. 'This morning, I was the devil incarnate.' He winks at you and begins walking into the ward, whistling, jangling keys. 'Hope you're feeling energetic. We've got a busy morning ahead.'

'Can't wait,' you lie.

'Communal lounge is here,' he says, pointing out rooms like a tour guide. 'Nursing station there. Male rooms up to the left. Females, right.' He puts a palm-sized plastic cylinder into your hand with a button at the top. You look at it as if it's a bomb.

'Panic alarm,' he says. 'Keep it with you at all times. You shouldn't have to use it.'

Before you can say anything, he's walking away. You squeeze the alarm, caress the button like the trigger of a gun, and follow.

'The ward is staffed by a multidisciplinary team,' Paul says. 'Each of us has our photo up here.' He points at a wall display, headshots of staff members. Top of the tree is the consultant psychiatrist.

'Dr Grace,' Paul says. 'She's the clinician responsible for all the patients.'

Psychiatrists like Dr Grace are medically trained, experts in the diagnosis and treatment of mental health conditions. Psychologists will have undertaken specialist research-informed training, usually to doctorate level, in one of the many forms of applied psychology, which is integrated into clinical practice. Psychotherapists will have undertaken extensive training too, including hours of personal therapy, to practise as registered talking therapists. All have psych in their title. And all do distinct roles.

Below Dr Grace there's a collaborative of highly trained professionals from a breadth of backgrounds – occupational therapy, social work, speech and language therapy, pharmacy and, of course, the mental health nurses like Paul, the blue-collar workers who do the heavy lifting and who make up the bulk of the psychiatric workforce.

According to a recent Statista Report, in late 2022 there were nearly 39,000 registered mental health nurses (RMNs) employed by the NHS. Most work on wards like this one, but you'll also find us in community teams, prisons, care homes, schools, local authorities, in the independent sector too, at private mental health care providers. And given the sharp spike in mental health difficulties the past few decades have seen, we're not likely to be out of work any time soon.

Traditionally, the role of the nurse in a mental health setting was custodial. 'Attenders', as they were known, were paid to run the asylums, their priority to keep the insane away from the public, a way to maintain the social order and remove those who deviated from it. But in the early twentieth century, 'mental nurse' became an official title, with the setting up of the Register for Mental Health Nurses under the General Nursing Council. Suddenly we had a role affiliated with clinical skills – caring, not judging, as the sign outside this ward read.

'C'mon,' Paul says, and you turn right, moving up a hall branching towards the lounge. You're sure you hear Emily howling again, from somewhere far off.

Posters are masking-taped to walls – Samaritans, Mental Health advocacy groups, men's groups, women's groups, LGBTQI+ groups, Care Quality Commission steering groups – peeling away from the plasterwork like dried skin.

The lounge is an open-plan space with heavy fire-retardant armchairs and a wall-mounted TV boxed in a Perspex cage. There are also patients here. Two men are slumped in armchairs. Both are shoeless. They wear loose T-shirts, hospital pants and furtive stares. In front of them stands a bald, bearded man in soiled jeans and an England top. His small eyes are enthralled by the TV, where a rerun of an antiques show plays, the volume low, like elevator muzak. As David Dickinson holds a ceramic teapot up at the camera, the bald man begins laughing.

'Every room here has a designated function,' Paul says, 'and when not used for that, it will make do for something else.'

'Where are we headed?' you ask.

'Group meeting room. Kelvin's being discussed. Have your hanky ready.' You're about to ask why, but Paul has stopped outside an anonymous door; he taps three times, enters. You follow him in.

It's a cramped, unremarkable office space. Brown felt armchairs in a horseshoe configuration, lilac wallpaper, a faded van Gogh print hung crookedly. You shut the door, aware of a fetid, beef-stock smell.

Dr Grace, the psychiatrist you recognise from her photo, sits at the head. Expensive heels, insistent perfume, a sensible smile. Beside her sits a heavily pierced woman whose lanyard identifies her as a staff nurse, Rose. Rose's eyes are glued to a laptop, her shellac nails clickety-clicking the keys. Beside Rose, there's an empty seat, and beside that, the patient.

Kelvin is a thin, middle-aged African-Caribbean man, and the source of the smell. He's dressed in tatty Reeboks, tracksuit bottoms, an oversized blazer; he has a flat cap pulled down, masking his eyes but revealing a face that resembles a crumpled tissue, with divots and nicks, flaky skin and white-headed pimples.

'Kelvin's being discharged later,' Paul says as the two of you sit down. 'Been here a week.'

'Congratulations, Kelvin,' you say.

Kelvin stares up at you, his bottom lip quivering like a plucked guitar string.

'Kelvin,' Dr Grace says, 'how're you feeling about leaving?'

Kelvin is silent.

'Kelvin?' she says.

Nothing.

'Your flat is ready. The council's changed the locks, cleaned it all up and—'

'Out there's not safe.' His voice is both gruff yet infantile, like a child raised on Marlboros. 'Can't I stay a bit longer?'

Why would anyone want to stay in this place? It seems insane. But Kelvin is serious.

Dr Grace adopts an expression: part sympathy, part pragmatism, no bullshit. 'You have a home,' she says. 'We've done all we can. But this isn't the right place for you.'

He inhales. 'Please,' he whispers, exhaling a stale breath, exposing a maw of yellowed teeth. Then he looks at you. 'Please.'

Paul clears his throat. Rose stops typing. Dr Grace sighs.

In any given town in the UK there will be Kelvins: oddballs, laughed at, pitied, avoided; they're vulnerable, lonely, just about getting by; they're like stray dogs scavenging – you feel sorry, but don't want to get too close.

Over the years, Kelvin has been passed around mental health services, housing services, social care services, voluntary aid services, everyone doing their best but failing to fix the problem fully. For what Kelvin needs is a community, people to look out for him, to check in, have him over for his tea. Instead, he has no one. He befriends undesirables – users, dealers, predators, fair-weather friends who hijack his flat and turn it into a squat.

Kelvin has foetal alcohol syndrome, a by-product of his late mother's alcoholism, causing him to have cognitive difficulties and autistic traits. He is vulnerable; but being on a mental health ward hasn't altered that vulnerability. It's merely caused his dependence.

His admission came about a week ago when police raided his flat that had been turned into a crack house. They quickly realised Kelvin had been cuckooed by county lines dealers who'd manipulated him.

After boarding up the flat as a crime scene, the police deposited Kelvin at A&E, then left. Before long, he was wailing and headbanging in the reception area. Unsure what to do, the nurses called in a mental health team, who were equally flummoxed. Kelvin had nowhere to go. They found him a bed on a mental health ward, the only place of safety they could think of. Here, he's grown dependent on the staff and safety he feels. And he's just been told he's to lose it all and be sent back into the world.

'I'm sorry,' Dr Grace says.

Kelvin looks at her.

'You can't stay forever. You knew this would come.' He looks back at the floor, his expression like a lost war.

'We'll discharge you after lunch.'

You feel for Dr Grace. This is a tough call. The National Confidential Inquiry into Suicide and Safety in Mental Health 2020 found that 14 per cent of all patient suicides happened within three months of discharge from inpatient care. And there's a wealth of evidence to support the demographic higher risk of suicidality among single disadvantaged males. Kelvin would tick those boxes. But pushing against this is the reality that Kelvin is taking up a much-needed mental health bed.

Really, there should be a representative from adult social services here, an advocate from a charity, someone from the housing department, and a friend or family member – all here to help Kelvin's transition out of hospital, consider what support he might need, and to be there. But there's no one.

Kelvin's eyes water. His face scrunches up. The first tear careens down his cheek. You watch it plop to the floor like acid rain. You look at Paul, hoping he will offer something. He is quiet.

Rose, the staff nurse, says, 'How about we get you a bath, Kel? Maybe we can dig out some clothes too.' Kelvin rubs his nose, swallows. There's nothing more to say. Paul stands. You follow, and you leave the office as one.

As soon as the door is closed, you're on to Paul: 'Isn't there something else you can do for him?'

'This job is as much about knowing what you *can't* do as what you *can*. Understand?'

You shake your head.

'Come with me, then,' he says. 'You will.' He's already leading the way towards the women's rooms.

'Where are we going?' you ask, cantering to keep up.

'To see Nikki.' He stops outside the furthest room down the hall. 'She's on one-to-one.'

'What's that?'

'It means there's a nurse with her always. She's high risk.'

'Risk of what?'

'Suicide.'

'Why?'

Paul clears his throat and tells you. Prior to the admission, Nikki, a single mother of four, brought her youngest two into five different emergency departments with serious vomiting, hacking coughs, fatigue. There were no obvious reasons for these symptoms but tests showed abnormally high levels of insulin in each child, enough to kill – insulin of the kind Nikki used for her type 1 diabetes.

It turned out that over the past two years, Nikki had been creating sicknesses in herself and her kids, moving around the country, attending emergency departments, registering with reams of GPs, trying to get admitted.

'Jesus Christ,' you say.

Paul nods.

'She could've killed her kids.'

He nods again.

'How did she end up here?'

'A shrewd nurse called the police. Before they could arrest Nikki, she gave her kids a hefty dose of insulin, took one herself, and they all fell into comas. Thankfully, no one died. After a week in intensive care, she woke up and learned that her kids had been taken by social services and she was facing charges of attempted murder. She informed nurses of her plans to end her life, started tying ligatures all over the ward. Given this threat, and the media interest in her, she was sent here, where she's been the past three months, getting cared for.'

'Cared for?' You say it like a swear word, thinking the obvious – who'd want to care for her?

Paul says, 'No matter what people have done, when they come to a place like this they deserve to be taken care of. It's what we do.'

You take a moment, trying to digest what you've just heard. It lodges like a fishbone. 'What's wrong with her?'

'She's got the munchies.'

'Huh?'

Paul explains. Munchausen by Proxy – or Factitious Disorder, its less pejorative name – is a rare mental disorder that sees the sufferer falsify symptoms of illness in others. It is complex, misunderstood, dangerous, and provokes all kinds of feelings of shock and repugnance – including from those paid to provide care.

Paul seems unfazed. He says: 'To Nikki, making her kids ill is a way of making them need her. It's an attempt to fill a hole. For a while it worked. Now that she's here, separated from them, locked up, she's waking up to what she did.'

'But how could she do that?' you say. 'To her kids?'

Paul shrugs again – a mannerism you're getting used to. 'She's unwell.'

You wait for more. Nothing.

'Ready?'

Before you can answer, Paul taps the door.

You enter a neat, spartan room with two occupants in it. A gum-chewing nurse, Chelsea, according to her ID, sits on a plastic chair. Directly opposite her, a thirty-something woman is supine on a single bed, knees to her chest. Her dark hair is split and matted; she has a round, pimply, honest face. She doesn't look like a monster. In fact, she looks like the fed-up mum you bashed trolleys with at Tesco the other day. Pale, tired, unremarkable, wearing bunny slippers, tracksuit bottoms, a plain white tee.

'Hello, Nikki,' Paul says to her, and explains who you are. While he speaks, you take in the room. It's functional, like a bedsitter after a clean-up; although there's something strange here too.

After a moment, you see it. The whole space has been rendered 'suicide proof'. No sharp edges, no bedposts, jutting locks, no shower rails, hooked taps, exposed cables or pipes;

the window, showing out to a car park, has the glass set far back, well out of reach; the door hook is attached with a magnetic lock, designed to detach harmlessly if a heavy load is applied, while the door handles all curve downwards, so that any ligatures tied on will slide to the floor like water through a flume. It all lends the room a soft, dreamy, Dalí-esque feel, like a wax diorama melting on a stove.

You return to Nikki, your pulse beginning to club.

As Paul finishes talking, she takes you in. Suddenly, you are struck by those eyes: the whites are veined red, but the pupils are obsidian stones – black, unrepentant, the only sharp edges here.

'You're visiting a nut house?' she says, a light, smoker's voice.

You don't reply.

'How does it feel?'

'What do you mean?'

'Seeing me?'

'I . . .' you say. 'I don't know. How do you feel being here?'

She rubs her eyes with the balls of her palms. They come away wet. Nurse Chelsea's chewing goes up a notch; she offers Nikki a Kleenex, along with a mawkish smile.

'C'mon, Nikki,' she says. 'Say how *you* feel being here?'

'Feel?' Nikki sniffs a cruel laugh and looks at you again. 'How do you think I feel, dickhead?'

You start.

'Now now, Nikki,' Paul says. 'No need for that.'

Silence fills the room, heavy and stagnant, like a dying breath. 'They say I tried to kill my kids,' she whispers. 'You hear about that?'

You nod.

'You believe them?'

You don't answer.

'Course you do. You think I'm a psycho. Well, I love my kids. They need me.' She pauses. 'If I can't have them, that's it. There's no way back. That's how I feel. OK?'

Chelsea looks at us, offers a 'what can you do?' shrug.

'It's over,' Nikki says, more to herself than you.

You look at Paul. He shrugs too.

'Go,' Nikki says. 'I don't want to talk.' She curls onto her side on the bed, brings her knees to her chest and faces the wall.

Paul gestures for the door. You leave with relief, feeling claggy and unclean.

Out in the hallway, you ask him, 'Why didn't you say something?'

He smiles sadly. 'Sometimes there's nothing you can say.'

'She's going to kill herself, isn't she? If she gets out and can't get her kids back.'

'Maybe.'

'What can you do to help?'

'Try to support her. And try not to judge.'

'Caring, not judging,' you say, repeating the sign outside the ward.

'But we need to be aware of our limitations too. The chance of Nikki being reunited with her kids is negligible. If she gets discharged from here, she'll likely be arrested for attempted murder. In prison, mums who try to kill their kids aren't top of the popularity tree. If you were in her shoes, would you want to live?'

You look away. 'It's so bleak,' you say.

'Correct,' Paul says with a strange glee. 'You're learning.'

Onwards, towards the nursing station, past the bald man in the lounge, now with his shirt off and in a full-flight conversation with the people on TV. Paul shows you the dining room, four circular plastic tables and curving chairs; the adjoining kitchen, a galley space loaded with paper plates and plastic cutlery. Inside, an unhappy cook is reheating an unhappy cod-slush for lunch, the smells stale, fishy.

Paul shows you the sluice room where an industrial washer rumbles through cycles of dirty clothes and bedding – bled on, vomited on, crapped on, cried on. He shows you the activity room crammed with paperbacks and boardgames donated from benevolent trusts, most ripped and missing bits. He shows you the staffroom, a piddly galley space, the floor and sill cluttered with dirty mugs, caked Pot Noodle tubs and piles and piles of weeks-old papers and magazines.

It's disgusting, like a student's digs after finals week, and reeks of fried fish, old feet and cat food. A wall of overflowing lockers dominates one side of the room; a manky kettle and fridge containing out-of-date yogurt is adjacent, and a staff nurse sleeps in one of the easy chairs. As you leave, his right eye opens and zeros on you like a samurai's.

You check your watch. You've only been here an hour but already feel exhausted.

'OK?' Paul says.

You nod. What you'd like now is the chance to chat with him over a brew, discuss things. But he's not letting up. 'C'mon,' he says.

'Where next?' you say, hoping for something less gruelling than the last two patient encounters.

'Seclusion,' he says, smiling.

There's a plunging in your gut. Seclusion refers to the enforced removal of particularly disturbed patients deemed to be an immediate risk to others on the ward. Seclusion spaces will vary from place to place, with some modern, having private toilet facilities and access to TV, others a bare room on full display.

This seclusion room, located down a dead-end corridor, is a room within a room. It's a single-occupant space with padded walls and a thick Perspex divider separating staff and patient. A last-resort area and the nearest thing to *The Silence of the Lambs* you've seen.

'Abi's here at the moment,' Paul says as you enter. 'She's been with us loads of times. Right now, she's unsettled.'

'What do you mean?'

'Another manic episode. She was trying to hurt herself. Needed some restraint and time to come down.'

'What was she doing?'

'Cutting. Headbanging. Inserting. Then she broke a health care assistant's nose when they tried to stop her.'

'Inserting?'

Paul points to his nether regions. 'Sharps.'

Your lips suck against your clenched teeth.

'We've given her some meds, but we'll need to keep her here till they take effect and she calms down. It looks like she may've taken some street drugs too while she's been here. That won't have done her any good.'

It's common knowledge that illicit substances wreak

havoc in prisons and across the homeless population in the UK. But you had no idea they had infiltrated mental health wards too.

'Where'd she get the drugs from?' you say.

'Who knows? But it's a big problem. Some patients come in for what should be a brief admission, then end up staying months when they tamper with that rubbish. Let's hope Abi's not one of them. Poor thing.'

Poor thing, you think.

Abi is naked. She sits on the floor, back to the wall, knees tight to her chest, swaying back and forth, shivering. Her clothes are strewn on the floor; apart from a seatless toilet, they are the only objects in there with her. She's young, Caucasian, with dark hair and a petite, athletic frame; she's pretty, with sharp bone lines and fierce dark eyes. Her arms and legs are riven with scars, fresh, raw, grinning. Both her eyes have yellow-grey panda bruises, there are patches of hair missing from her scalp, and her lower lip swells like an amoeba.

She's under the gaze of two burly male nurses, both stood behind the glass, watchful.

'Why's she not got any clothes on?' Paul says.

'She keeps pulling them all off,' one of the nurses replies.

Paul shakes his head. 'She can't be exposed like that. Give her a towel, please. Make sure she doesn't try anything with it.'

The other nurse kisses his teeth, and they root in a drawer, pull out a bath towel, unlock the Perspex door, walk in side by side. Abi, scared and exposed, stares up at these two large, dressed men. The difference in power is stark. She takes the towel, wraps it over her shoulders like a gown.

As the nurses leave, you whisper to Paul, 'All those wounds on her. They're—'

'Self-inflicted,' he says. 'Yes. Of course.'

'But . . . why?' You look at him. 'Why would she do all this?'

'Abi has bipolar affective disorder,' he says. 'Unless she takes care of herself, accepting meds, engaging with her community mental health team, her moods get erratic and she ends up in a state like this.'

'What happened?'

'This time, she fell for the wrong bloke, decided to come off her meds because of the side-effects and started messing around with street drugs he gave her instead. Eventually he got bored, dumped her, and she went into a nosedive. Maxed out her credit cards shopping on Oxford Street. Copped off with random strangers. Took more drugs. Got picked up by the police in a phone booth wearing a blood-spattered fur coat, clutching a Chanel handbag full of cash, drugs and razors.'

It's like something out of a shock-horror comedy. But there's nothing funny about Abi.

You look at her again. She's spotted you now. Her eyes are wet and dirty, like two glasses of pond water. Tendons cord the skin of her neck like tree vines. Something calcifies in you.

'What's going to happen to her?' you ask.

'Right now,' Paul says, 'our job is to keep her and others on the ward safe till the meds we've given her kick in, and those she's taken leave her system. When she comes to, she'll be a different person. That's when the real work comes in.'

'Real work?'

'She'll find out what she's done, and she'll be riddled with shame.'

'Why?'

'She's burned bridges this time. Spending money she can't afford. Causing her disabled mum no end of worry. Mental illness is cruel. It pushes away the people you love.'

You step up to the partition, close enough for your breath to fog the glass. Abi stares. You stare back. Again, the power imbalance is profound. You feel self-conscious, like you're gazing at a scared animal in a zoo.

'C'mon,' Paul says. 'Clive's expecting us in the meds room about now.'

'Clive?' You scramble to keep up, for Paul is on the move again, leading you through the security doors, back through the corridor, out towards the communal lounge, stopping outside a door. A sign reads MEDICATION ROOM. He taps and steps in.

Two men are inside another narrow room. One is sitting, one standing; both are bald. You recognise them as the pair you passed earlier, headed out on escorted leave.

But something's wrong with this picture.

The tall man, still dressed for the office, is sitting on a stool, his back to the wall. The short man, unkempt, dishevelled, preps tablets from a trolley full of medication. An NHS lanyard hangs around his meaty neck, informing you that his name is Warren, and he's a staff nurse.

You feel surprise, then a bolt of shame hits like a cattle prod. You'd made assumptions about the pair, about which was the patient, which the clinician, based on how they looked. And you'd been wrong.

'Hello again,' the tall man on the stool says cheerily. 'I'm Clive. I gather you want to talk to some of us.'

You look at Paul. He nods. You enter the narrow room. Clive's tart aftershave strikes you, along with his beady eyes and winning smile. You can imagine him working a sensible nine to five job, driving a sensible Corsa, volunteering at church groups and posting jumble sale pamphlets through doors. Why's he on a ward with Nikki and Abi and all the others?

'I can read your mind,' he says.

'Huh?'

'You're wondering why I'm here?'

You nod.

'Where should I begin?'

You hesitate. 'Maybe say a bit about yourself. If that's OK?'

'I'll try,' he says. 'I'm fifty-one, a bachelor and a civil servant. I've worked for the council for twenty-three happy years. I love my job. Never missed a day . . .' He pauses: 'Until all this.'

'All this?'

He looks at Paul, behind you. 'They've been vetted?'

'Everything's fine, Clive,' Paul says. 'Remember what we talked about?'

Clive returns to you. 'I'm sorry. I don't mean to be rude, but you can't be too careful.'

'No problem.'

He smiles again. 'I started sleeping in the office. Under my desk. I'd have a shower in the local swimming pool each morning, go out for tea at a café, and then snuggle up once the cleaners had gone for the night. That way, I didn't have to go home.'

'Why didn't you want to go home?' you ask.

He smiles; this time, the smile twitches. 'The spies,' he whispers.

'Spies?'

His eyes flit left and right. 'They've been trying to get me. For years.'

You wait.

Clive says, 'If I tell you, do you promise not to go to the media?'

'I promise.'

'It could put you in grave danger.'

'You have my word.'

Satisfied, he starts. 'It's a strange story.'

And it is. For years, Clive has been struggling to evade the aforementioned spies, feeling their presence, spotting them in shadows, hearing them muttering, yet holding himself together at work, the only place where he found refuge.

'I call them spies but they're more like secret operatives. Russian mercenaries. Pagan cults. Sex perverts. Anarchists. I'm not entirely sure of their origin, but they're a global infrastructure. They formed an allegiance hell-bent on destroying civilisation and have been after me for years.'

'Why?' you ask.

'Because I'm the only person who knows who they are. They've come close to annihilating me, but I've outwitted them. So far, that is.' He licks his lips. A bead of sweat runs from his forehead.

'Easy, Clive,' Paul says from behind you.

Clive looks at him, nods. Then he returns to you.

'The staff here think I've got something wrong in my head.' He taps his brow again. 'You know, losing my marbles. But I know the truth. It's why I did what I did.'

'What you did?'

He tells you.

A week prior to this admission, Clive's manager told him she was concerned that he was spending so much time at work and suggested he take some time off. When he declined, she insisted. Clive was forced to return home to his little flat. With only his head for company, the fissures expanded. He became a frequent caller to the police and fire services, complaining of bugs in the walls and furniture, shadowy intruders trying to break in. He accused the neighbours of being assassins, blacked out his windows with bin sacks, blocked the chimney with rubble to keep safe.

'I even disowned my dotty old mum.'

'Why?' you say.

'The tone of her voice. The order of the words she used. It was a sign. I knew she was in on the conspiracy too.'

You nod, working to keep your face impassive while he tells the rest.

'It reached boiling point four days ago. In the middle of the night, I woke to a scratching. It was like a radio stuck between stations. Straightaway, I knew what was happening.'

'What?'

'They'd managed to surgically implant a microchip into my brain.'

'Oh.'

'Of course, I had to act. If I didn't, lives could be lost.'

And act he did. That same night, Clive attempted to steal an MRI scanner from his local hospital, planning to pinpoint the exact location in his cranium where the chip had been fitted. He would then remove it with a selection of garden tools he'd stolen from a neighbour's shed.

Your poker face cracks, for you're sure he's exaggerating. But the stark look in Clive's eyes tells you he's serious: he would've followed through, quite possibly killing himself in the process.

'But I got pipped to the post,' he says. 'The hospital security spotted me. Said I was acting strangely. They called the police. I was arrested, and when I told police why I had to steal the MRI, and why I had a backpack of tools, they brought me here.'

'What about the microchip?' you say.

He nods, smiles. 'It's still in me.'

You want to ask more, but the short nurse hands Clive a small paper tub of pills. 'Here you go, Clive,' he says, his voice infused with gruff kindness.

Clive inspects the pills, tilting his head side to side, viewing them forensically. You know what he's thinking – they're bugged too, implanted with more microchips. After a long minute, he knocks them back with a glug of water, swallows, and shuts his eyes. When they open, he looks at you.

'Do you think I'm crazy?'

You're struck silent.

Imagine it, to be told that the belief you held prescient for years is a delusion. Part of Clive is clinging onto the certainty that there are spies conspiring against him. But another part is coming round to the cruel truth that his mind is the enemy.

You say, 'I think what you've experienced is real for you.' This isn't the first time Clive has heard this, or phrases like it. In confirmation, he gives you one of the saddest smiles you've seen.

'What a horrid mess,' he says. 'If you wouldn't mind, I'd like to be alone now.'

You step outside.

Paul shuts the door, says, 'You're getting good at this.'

You look at him, shocked. 'What do you mean?'

'I mean, you're learning when to ask questions. And when not to.' While you're mulling this over, Paul checks his watch. Warm food smells waft around the ward, and there's the clang of pots and pans.

'It's lunchtime soon,' he says. 'Protected time. Visitors must leave, I'm afraid. But there's one more thing to see first.' You follow him to the nursing station, positioned central to the ward. 'It's the nerve centre.' He swipes you in with his key fob. 'We're about to have a quick MDT.'

'MDT?'

Multi-disciplinary team meeting, Paul explains, another abbreviation, refers to the gathering of the different professionals that make up the workforce. 'So that we're up to speed with challenges, and all on the same page.'

You're expecting a well-oiled conference, maybe with handouts and slides. Instead, Paul takes you into a cluttered, claustrophobic, uncomfortably warm room. A thick glass wall offers a panoptical view of the patients' lounge; everything else is machines and bodies.

There's half a dozen staff here – nurses, doctors, typing, on calls, making notes in files; there's three aged desktop computers, a printer, alarm panels, phones, humming and beeping and droning atonally; on every chair hangs a coat, on every inch of desk lies a folder; plastic boxes sit beneath the desks containing lighters, phone cables, cigarettes, contraband removed from patients; beside these, Health and Safety folders, Prevention of Violence and Aggression folders, Mental Health Act folders, and reams and reams more.

A box of Jaffa Cakes spills out over a thick file of papers stapled together. When you read the heading, you see it's an inquest report.

'A quick word about EH,' Paul says, standing by a whiteboard on the wall. This board lists all the patients denoted by initials, room number, diagnoses and whether they're sectioned or not. EH, you realise, refers to Emily, the screamer you met on your way in.

'She's been vocal today,' Paul says. 'Tried her Houdini escape trick earlier.'

'She's on intermittent obs,' the nurse says. 'Why don't we give her thirty minutes escorted leave to the shops and see how she gets on?'

No one speaks.

The nurse looks at Paul. 'I gather you've got a special relationship with Emily. Fancy a jaunt out?'

'Can't wait,' he says, scowling. His colleagues chuckle. 'Next, there's NB. Currently on one-to-one. How's she doing, Chelsea?'

NB, of course, is Nikki.

Chelsea, the gum-chewing nurse from earlier, picks up

a clipboard, reads, 'Still saying the same thing: if she can't get her kids back, she'll top herself. Police called again this morning, asking when they can interview her for attempted murder.' Chelsea lowers the clipboard, blows a bubble that inflates and pops over her mouth like an abrupt full stop.

'She's high risk,' Paul says, his expression grave, to murmurs of agreement. 'If the police call again, tell them she's not fit for interview any time soon. If they give you grief, put them onto me.'

Next, they discuss Abi, still in seclusion, still naked, still agitated.

'She's been there four hours now,' someone says. 'Whatever drugs she's taken have really pushed her over the edge.'

'Rapid tranqs were given at the start of shift,' Paul says. 'There's been little benefit. She's a tough girl. Refuses to put her clothes back on.'

'She keeps trying to put stuff into her noo-noo,' someone else adds.

You're not sure what shocks you more: the graphic imagery of this disturbed young woman's sexual sadomasochism or the chuckles that this last remark provoke.

Paul turns to Dr Grace, sitting in the corner.

'Can you write her up for something stronger?'

Dr Grace fishes out a gnarled prescription pad, starts scribing a higher dose of fast-active sedatives with one hand, reaching for a Jaffa Cake with the other.

They carry on this way, moving down the board, discussing each patient by their initials, their symptoms, their behaviour. It's dehumanising and, in its own way, as disturbing as everything else you've witnessed. But you're beginning to understand that it isn't callousness, or a sign that these men and women have stopped caring. It's a survival technique. Without gallows humour, the bleakness would overwhelm. For in this ward, the abhorrent, the abnormal, are as familiar as the Jaffa Cakes Dr Grace is munching.

A thud on the window makes you jump. No one else flinches. It's the TV talking man banging the glass. His eyes are wide.

'Lunch,' he shouts.

'We better get out there,' Paul says. 'Before we do, there's Kelvin. He's finally been given his marching orders.'

'I saw to it he got a bath,' says Rose, the nurse from Kelvin's ward round. 'Dug him out some new clothes. Gave him sommat to eat. He wants to stay.'

'Poor bugger,' someone says. 'Couldn't we keep him till tomorrow?'

'Bed management need his room pronto,' Paul says. 'I'll see him out. Along with our latest addition.' He looks directly at you. 'How've you got on?'

Your lungs fill with lead.

'I . . .' you say, then flounder. 'It's been good. Really good, thanks.' At this, the whole room laughs.

As Paul leads you from the nursing station towards the entrance, you see patients congregating in the dining area, tucking into reheated packaged meals spooned onto plastic receptacles like baby food. For a moment you take them in as one. They are unique, incongruous yet strangely aligned, like a crew of extras who've all turned up to the wrong film set. There's Nikki, sitting alone, spooning mash around a bowl. There's Clive, inspecting each mouthful of his fish mornay for bugs. There's Emily, eating just a bowl of gloopy custard, her eyes wide and hawkish. And there's Kelvin, finishing a ham sandwich, a bag of clothes by his side.

There are others too – a man in a wheelchair, military regalia pinned to his soiled blazer; a gangly Asian man, his hair a buzz cut, eyebrows shaved; a gaunt, gender-ambiguous twenty-something wearing a pink dressing gown, DM boots and a mirthless smile; a thin, bearded, long-haired Jesus lookalike making the sign of the cross.

Each has a backstory. And an uncertain future ahead.

At one point, Emily's eyes widen. She looks around like a startled cat. You're sure she's about to start her screaming again. Instead, Kelvin walks up and places a hand on hers.

'There there, Em.' You see him mouth the words. She looks at him, rattled. Then relief flows into her. She returns to her custard and you exhale a breath you hadn't realised you'd been holding.

'Ready, Kelvin?' Paul says.

Kelvin nods and stands. He's wearing a too-big Umbro tracksuit and Hush Puppies without socks. But the pungent smell from before is gone. The three of you walk to the main entrance you came through, the backdrop of chatter fading out. No one speaks. At the door, you hand the panic alarm back to Paul.

'Said you wouldn't need it,' he says.

You smile. But the smile fades when you see Kelvin, shuffling on the spot. Paul holds his fob to the door reader. It thuds open. You hold it ajar.

As Kelvin passes through, Paul says, 'I hope I don't see you again.'

You look back, but he's already turned, and the door to the ward is shut.

You walk with Kelvin, back through the hallways you came in by, and then exit the hospital. Outside, the lunchtime sky is bold and insistent, and you feel glad to be free. Kelvin doesn't seem aware. He asks if you'd like to go with him to McDonald's, offers to buy you a McFlurry. You decline. You don't fancy sitting in McDonald's. And you don't fancy sitting opposite Kelvin, trying to think of things to say.

Back home, you are quick to return to who you were. Cooking. TV. Socials. But that evening you find yourself showering longer than normal, scrubbing your fingertips, rinsing your hair twice over. As you towel down, you think about Abi, naked in that seclusion room, and wonder if she's still there. You think about Emily, stood by the entrance, desperate to escape. You think about Kelvin, eating his McFlurry alone, desperate to go back.

You tell yourself that a mental health ward is a sad reality of life, but a necessity too. At the very least, today's visit will provide you with a story or two to tell your friends. You try to switch off with this.

But you can't.

You're struck by how care of the mentally ill is a nuanced job, as much about metaphor and politics, phenomenology and ethics as it is about anatomy and physiology, diagnoses and drugs. Sometimes it's about combinations of treatment, or close-up observations of behaviour; other times it's about the tone of voice, a gentle touch, the gaps between words. You're disturbed by what you saw. But you're moved, too.

Paul's parting words catapult back: *I hope I don't see you again.* Perhaps it was meant for Kelvin, a glib way to encourage him to keep himself well, move forward and not return. But perhaps it was meant for you too.

Maybe you hope you don't see the ward again either. You want to close the book, gawp at Insta food porn and ephemeral holiday snaps, go to bed and forget. Fair enough.

Maybe you're exhausted from today, thankful to have had the opportunity to see what goes on in these maligned, misunderstood places, but tomorrow you're ready for something new. Fair enough too.

Or maybe you feel the way I did after my visit to a mental health ward. The electromagnetic door thuds, the salty tears, harsh screams and desperate laughs seep back into your consciousness, meshing into a tableau. You get to sleep in the small hours, but it isn't restful. You wake, realising that a swathe of feeling has filled you, vast and heady, yours to carry. It's as if a plaster has been ripped off, exposing a wound that has always been there, but unnoticed until now, and leaves you with an angry sadness.

I hope I don't see you again.

If only it were true.

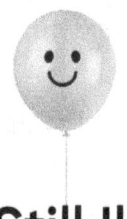

Still Ill

'Hi, Samir,' I say. 'I'm Elliot. A trainee nurse. I'm going to give you your injection today. Have a seat.'

Samir remains standing by the clinic room door. His arms are folded; he's scrutinising me. 'My name's Sam, not Samir,' he says, his tone all street edge and London. 'You're a student?'

I flash the student ID around my neck, smile.

'Fuck off.'

Sam's as tall as me but broader, stockier, dominating the small room we're in like an Alsatian in a cot. He's wearing oxblood DMs, distressed denim, a T-shirt that says, 'The Voices Made Me Do It', and has a pink-rose-leafed bandana on his scalp. His skin is a milky tea colour, his chin dusted with wispy black hairs, and his eyes rarely blink, but instead hold me in exactitude, like a rancher staring at a pig on abattoir day.

'Relax,' I say. 'I may be a student but I know what I'm doing.'

Scorn wafts from Sam like an oven door left open. I turn to the counter, begin preparing his fortnightly injection of antipsychotic medication, my eyes flitting between the textbook in front of me and the apparatus I've assembled.

I'm halfway into my training now. Administering an intramuscular injection – known as a depot – is a mandatory requirement for us students if we want to pass the diploma. I've practised on grapefruits and oranges, mimed the stretching out of the target area with one hand, drawing back the syringe like a dart before firing; I've mastered aspirating the plunger, ensuring no veins or arteries have been hit, applying slow, steady pressure until the solution is all in. I'm ready – all that's needed is for me to practise on a real-life human.

It's mid-July, one of those savage London summers, and we're within a community mental health team base in central London. Rather than a purpose-built building, the team base occupies a third of a complex, the other two-thirds comprising a graphic design start-up and a wealth management consortium. The conversations that take place in the shared toilets between mental health patients, arty hipsters and corporate suits scale a new height of strange.

This clinic room is set in the bowels of the building adjacent to the grumbling generators. It's an enclosed space. There's a drugs cabinet, a work surface, a chair, a gurney and an opaque window looking out onto a brick wall. The lack of ventilation, the proximity of machines, furniture, bodies, makes the heat punishing, and beads of perspiration run over my brow.

'You're sweating,' Sam says.

'It's hot,' I say, and wipe my brow.

'You nervous?'

'No.'

'He's fine,' Alan, my mentor, says from the corner of the room. 'Relax, Sam.'

I glance over, lock eyes with Alan, who gives a reassuring nod. Alan, who encouraged me into mental health nursing, came to the job after falling homeless. He has the scars, demeanour, the droll humour to show for it. For the past few weeks I've shadowed him in all aspects of his role as a community mental health nurse, and he pre-warned me about Sam, one of the more challenging patients.

Presently, Sam is staring at the unctuous solutions I've drawn through a needle into a large syringe. This is a slow-release drug called flupentixol decanoate, designed to dampen the voices Sam hears because of his schizophrenia.

'If he's fine,' Sam says to Alan, 'why's he got that textbook with him? And why's he looking so green?'

'I'm not green,' I say, and snap the book shut. Sam mutters something I don't make out.

Ignoring the tethering in my gut, I survey my kit a final time, imagining myself like a surgeon with his scalpels: there's the syringe, the alcohol rub, the elastic plaster. Next to these is Sam's medication chart.

Behind me, Sam carries on muttering. This is one of his symptoms – 'responding' – meaning he's having a natter with people we can't see. I ignore the sound, focus on my task at hand. Even so, words jump out – 'numpty student'; 'speccy idiot'; 'guy's got a lot to learn'. My hands begin to tremble.

'Hey,' Sam says abruptly. I turn too fast, elbowing my textbook off the counter. It clunks to the floor.

'What?' I say. Streams of sweat careen down my neck and chest, darkening my shirt.

'You've done this before, right?' he says.

'I've practised,' I assure him, and add, 'don't worry, you won't feel a thing.' Sam doesn't answer, but his lips keep moving and his stare is unwavering.

In general, patients are put onto a depot when taking tablets isn't working out. For some, remembering to take a pill daily is too much for them to manage; for others, there is an aversion to taking mental health meds in general, and this is the only way of ensuring they receive what's prescribed.

Sam falls into this camp. If he swerves the fortnightly injection he could be recalled to hospital, where he'll be restrained and given the medication by force. Sam, for good reasons, isn't happy.

'I'm not happy,' he says.

'Why's that?' I ask.

'I don't like that stuff.' He points at the syringe.

'What don't you like about it?'

'How'd you feel if a stranger jabbed you in the arse every fortnight with chemicals?'

I take a moment. 'I'd feel annoyed.'

Sam hesitates. I've made a dint. 'What do you know, Florence Nightingale?' he mutters, and the guard returns.

What do I know? This past year, I've swapped Chandler and Hammett for dense books on psychopathology and the aetiology of mental disorder. I can talk shop about dopamine models of psychosis, schizophrenogenic parenting, the impact of socioeconomics and stigma. I'd love to tell Sam about all this, explain exactly what's wrong in his head. But he doesn't seem keen. Especially with me.

I return to my task, comparing the drug I'm about to give with Sam's medication chart. This is basic nursing. Right patient – check. Right medication – check. Right time – check. Right dose – check. Right route of administration – check.

I look at Alan. Another nod.

'OK,' I say. 'Ready?'

'Just get this over with,' Sam snarls, his mouth like a gash in a piece of bad fruit.

The favoured place for depots is the upper-outer gluteal, that dense meaty muscle beneath subcutaneous fat located on the buttock. Sam unbuckles his jeans belt, lowers the hem, and then pulls his boxers down to his groin, exposing a sizable chunk of flesh. The skin has been injected into many times and looks hard, cratered, heavily scarred.

Saying nothing, he lies on the gurney bed, chin on the mattress, hands at his side. I approach, place the injection equipment on a side table. Sam watches my every move. I pull gloves from a dispenser and plunge my hands into the latex. The sweat on my palms makes the skin stick, and two fingers on my right hand tear through the thin material.

'Clumsy,' Sam says.

Now my cheeks are a conflagration.

'No bother,' Alan says. 'Happens to us all.'

I peel the glove off, deposit it in the clinical waste bin, remove another set.

'Chop, chop,' Sam says. 'Got places to be.'

My mouth twitches. Carefully, I insert my hand, each digit slotting into place neatly. Then I take the syringe and step up to the gurney, hovering over Sam's behind. His exposed buttock is like a landing pad. His still, dark eyes bale at me.

I visualise drawing a cross on the skin, then another cross within the top-right box, the upper-outer zone. I pinpoint a dot marked in the skin, next to a mole. This is where I will insert the needle. I look at Alan, point to this area. Nod.

Syringe ready, I place my hand on Sam's skin. He tenses. Gently, I stretch taut the skin with thumb and finger. It whitens.

'OK?' I say.

'Just do it.'

The syringe is huge, a .44 magnum, locked and loaded. *Do you feel lucky, punk?*

I pull back my wrist, inhale . . .

'Sharp scratch . . .'

Then I fire.

Many times I've gone over what went wrong. Perhaps Sam coughed or jerked; perhaps I slipped, or mistargeted? I still can't really explain it. Whatever, I know immediately that I've messed up. A steamy belch of shame pumps through me. And then my right hand starts to throb something awful.

This is bad. Really bad. Worse than the time I barged over a blind kid as I was rushing to catch a bus; worse than the time I asked a female friend who'd put on a few pounds when the baby was due.

I haven't injected Sam. The needle has impaled the loose

flap of skin between my thumb and finger, going deep, very deep into me. I've stabbed myself.

'Everything all right?' Sam says.

The blue glove sheathed over my right hand fills with red, as if claret is being drip-fed into the latex. I look over at Alan. My breath rasps. My vision fogs. I feel sick and want to run. But I can't run. Because I've got a patient lying prone and a syringe loaded with antipsychotics nailed into me.

'Oh,' Alan says, stepping over, looking at my hand. 'Whoops.'

'M-made a mistake,' I stutter.

'What mistake?' Sam says. 'The hell you done, student?'

'Nothing, Sam,' Alan says. 'Relax.'

Dark thoughts plunge into my head. What if I'm stuck this way forever? What if some of the meds have entered my bloodstream?

With my left hand I grip my wrist and step away from Sam. The syringe wobbles like a tent peg in the wind but stays rooted. I shuffle towards the medication cabinet. The glove is saggy with blood. I feel sick. I want the floor to eat me.

'Easy,' Alan says, stood beside me. Carefully, he holds the top of the syringe between thumb and finger and then pulls.

'Aah,' I say, as the metal slithers out, ending with a pool of fresh blood spilling from the latex. My knees are shaking. My mouth tastes of warm Parmesan.

Alan disposes of the syringe in a sharps bin. 'Run some cold water over it,' he says.

I peel the glove off, hold my hand beneath the flowing tap, watch my blood dilute and swirl down the sink.

The hole is small, a perfect circle from which a beautiful blossom of spidery red keeps appearing.

'Am I going to–'

'You'll be fine,' Alan says. 'You'll need to get a tetanus. Write an incident report. And you won't do that again, aye?'

I grab a paper towel from the dispenser, squeeze the wound hard. Gradually, the bleeding stops. I look over at Sam. He's now sitting up on the gurney, his jeans pulled back up, his lips muttering again. Between words, a toothy grin stretches across his mouth, and his eyes light up for the first time.

'You were right,' he says. My expression must show my confusion.

'I never felt a thing.' He begins laughing.

Pride sizzles in my guts like a rasher of bacon hitting the pan. I look at Alan for support but he's turned away, his shoulders juddering.

'It's not funny,' I say, and laugh too.

Suffice to say I failed the injection module of the course.

After getting a tetanus jab, and then enduring the indignity of a management debrief about what went wrong, I was given the green light to return to my training for another stab, pun intended. By then, any bemusement about what happened had worn thin.

It wasn't just the experience of stabbing myself that had jaded me. Earlier that year, during an inpatient placement, I'd witnessed a barbaric restraint and enforced treatment – four burly nurses rugby-tackling a sexually traumatised woman while a fifth administered a rapid tranquiliser into her posterior; I'd seen a young female health care assistant get battered by a dementia patient, her eyes like cut nectarine flesh by the end of the ordeal; I'd overheard pejorative, crude, demonising and foul language dished out by seasoned nurses about patients they were paid to care for; seen sloppy record keeping, gross fabrications, incompetent communication, flagrant disregard and general meanness; and, of course, there was Jack's suicide, still simmering.

The Nursing and Midwifery Council, the body that registers all nurses in the UK, requires nurses of all disciplines to adhere to four overarching themes: prioritise people, practise effectively, preserve safety and promote professionalism and trust. Each sounds clear-cut, but when you're in the eye of the storm, it's a little more complex. I was beginning to wonder if I was cut out for this gig.

The two-year diploma course had been sold as a blended form of learning, part classroom based, part placements within the NHS, the dual elements complementing one another in harmony.

The reality was quite different, and invariably felt ramshackle and shoddy. Lecturers didn't turn up, taught erroneous information, and a few appeared to have mental health issues themselves; placements collapsed, with mentors leaving, managers having meltdowns and students being asked to plug staff shortages and carry out dangerous tasks they weren't qualified to perform. It left a sour taste, and I wasn't the only one with doubts. Others in my cohort dropped out, frustrated and demoralised.

Looking back now, I can see it wasn't all bad. Compared

with today's student nurses, we weren't forced to rack up thousands of pounds of debt in course fees, and instead were paid a modest salary to train. We were also pretty much guaranteed a job post-completion, largely due to the national shortage of mental health nurses keen to work in the UK. Those of us who stuck with it were able to forge alliances, sharing horror stories, comedy ones, thawing out at the uni bar over games of pool.

Even so, it often felt gruelling – a dirty, dingy business – and seemed altogether quite bleak. When I compared myself to friends from school donning starched shirts and heading for internships in the city, I'd ask myself – why am I doing this? Why not get a 'normal' job?

This pessimism takes an unexpected turn a couple of weeks after the hand-impaling incident. I'm with Alan in a side room at the community mental health team base, looking over some notes, when he slams me with two bits of information.

'So,' he says, with an air of apology, 'I've got to go have a wee bit of chemo.'

'Chemo?' I say, then I add, gormlessly, 'Why?'

'Why do you think?'

I stare.

'I shouldn't be gone too long. Depends how it goes.'

'Yes,' I say. 'Right.'

'But it means my patients will have to be divvied out. While I'm away, someone has to keep an eye on them. And one of my favourites said he'd like you to swing by.'

My mind, still numb, flits down the list of Alan's cases. I've got to know most of the thirty-seven patients. I've formed a rapport with a few of the older ladies he sees, and suspect it's one of them.

'Who?' I ask.

Despite the waxy skin and yellow tinge to Alan's eyes, which makes sense now, he gives a wry smile and tells me.

'Sam?' I say, shock mingling with discomfort.

'Take it as a compliment,' Alan says. 'Sam's a hard nut to crack. He said the only person he'd be willing to see is that trainee who stabbed himself.'

'But . . . why?'

'Maybe he liked what he saw.'

'But I bodged things.'

'Exactly.' Alan chuckles, which turns into a raking cough.

To begin, I scrutinise Sam's notes. They're full of clinical jargon, acronyms and abbreviations, describing medication lists, detentions to hospital, working diagnoses, established diagnoses, treatment plans, revised treatment plans. It's all problem-focused, pathological and dehumanising stuff. Key terms lurch out – treatment-resistant schizophrenia; persecutory ideas; non-engaging with clinical staff; oppositional personality.

Oppositional. That much I can buy.

At first, Sam and I exchange texts. They go something like this:

Me: Hi Sam, this is Elliot, from the mental health team. How are you today?

Sam: Fine.

Me: That's good. Are you ready to meet up?

Sam: No.
A little later:
Me: Hi Sam, me again. Anything I can do?
Sam: No.
A little after that, my phone rings. Sam's voice: 'Let's meet up now.'

We go for coffee. An Italian café near Sam's flat in Kentish Town where there's outside seating beneath the awning where he can smoke.

Sam's as striking, and as strange, as the man I remember, clad in distressed denim, DMs, a flowery T-shirt and the same pink-rose bandana from last time. He carries a distinctive scent, part dense perfume fused with a gamy body smell. His fingers are slight, nicotine-stained, the cuticles picked, nails bitten to the quick. When he lifts the cigarette, his lips mutter, silently, wordlessly, as if recounting a song.

'So,' I say.

He looks at me, a shoot-from-the-hip glare.

'How are you, Sam?'

Silence.

'Alan sends his best.'

'Is he dead?'

'No. He's doing OK.'

'He could die, though.'

'I hope not.'

Sam considers me through a curd of smoke. He says, 'You're still nervous.'

I shrug.

'Were you embarrassed? After what happened?'

I remember the sight of my impaled hand, and Sam lying

with his jeans and pants by his ankles, laughing. Suddenly, I'm glad we're seated outside, for my cheeks are cooled by a slight breeze.

'Yes,' I say, 'I was embarrassed. That was a bad day.'

'Takes it out of you,' he says, 'being exposed. Don't you think?'

I indicate it does.

'You like your course?'

'Not particularly.'

'So why've you stuck at it?'

'I guess I don't like giving up on things.'

'That why you're here with me? 'Cause you don't want to give up?'

'Maybe,' I say. It feels like I'm being tested. Right now, I'm dejected enough not to care.

He carries on smoking, and for a moment he vanishes in the haze. When he reappears, I notice he's locked onto a paperback in my pocket, a thumbed Penguin Classic of *The Big Sleep*.

'You like that book?' he asks.

I shrug. 'Kind of.' A pause. 'Do you?'

'Not one of his best. The plot's woolly, but the dialogue is good.'

I'm surprised. Impressed too.

'What,' Sam says, 'you think schizophrenics can't read?'

'I–'

He sniggers, and for the first time his eyes light up. 'I'm going now,' he says, and stands abruptly.

'Hold up,' I say, staring at him. 'What do we–'

'Same time next week,' he says, and wanders off, leaving

a soldering cigarette in the ashtray, an unpaid bill for me to pay, and a pile of questions for me to contend with.

We carry on this way, meeting for coffee, Sam taking the lead, asking the questions. In exchange he allows me, under supervision, to practise a second intramuscular injection on his rear. This time, lo and behold, I get it right.

I probably tell him more than I should – about my home life, my partner Clare, our plans to travel, tie the knot; I tell him I was in a band when I was younger, played at the Bull and Gate up the road from where he lives.

He nods pensively. It's Sam's turn to be impressed.

'Here,' he says one afternoon, pulling an A3 pastel sketch from a satchel. We're at our usual spot outside the café in Kentish Town. We're regular enough for the waitress to know how we take our coffees, and that I'm the one who foots the bill.

I stare down at the drawing Sam unfurls. It depicts a trenchcoated figure stood on a desolate street corner, smoking beneath a dimly lit lamppost. In bold at the head of the sheet are the words, 'The Big Sleep'. Sam's depicted a front cover of the book I'd been reading.

'You did that?'

'Yeah.'

'You're good.'

'No, I'm not.'

The waitress appears with our drinks. Sam removes the artwork, making space on the table. She's clearly impressed too.

'See,' I say, gesturing at her. 'You're talented.'

There's a flush of colour to Sam's cheeks. 'I'm putting

work together for my portfolio. I want to go to art school.'

'Wow,' I say. I had no idea.

Sam, I learn, is drawn to all things creative, especially when the subject matter veers towards the darker realms of life. Despite the interruptions caused by his mental ill health and admissions, he's a prolific painter, sketcher, portraitist, cartoonist. I tell him about my own dalliances with creative writing, how I'm sure I have a book in me. As we speak, it dawns on me that I could be talking to any art student in London who takes themselves a little too seriously.

Only Sam's not that. He's a patient. A schizophrenic.

According to NICE, schizophrenia affects approximately fourteen and a half people in every thousand in the UK. Chances are you'll have brushed shoulders with a schizophrenic in the supermarket, boarding a bus, in GP surgeries, train stations, pubs, raves, soft-play centres with your kids.

Defining schizophrenia is the task of a psychiatrist, trained to use diagnostic skills to pinpoint a constellation of symptoms. Although there are varying sub-types of the illness, these symptoms can broadly be separated into two camps: positive and negative.

Positive symptoms refer to those that typically add something abnormal to the sufferer: auditory, visual, olfactory or tactile hallucinations, feelings of persecution, paranoia, grandiose or bizarre beliefs with no basis in reality. Negative symptoms refer to those that strip the sufferer of something they once had: a decline in self-care, impoverished speech, loss of interest and drive, blunted affect, a generalised apathy and disregard for things.

Schizophrenia is *not* split personality, and it has *nothing* to do with psychopathic behaviour: statistically, those with the illness pose more risk to themselves than others; and they are more likely to fall victim to abuse and discrimination than they are to be perpetrators. Yet to be a schizophrenic means carrying a spiky sack of pejoratives and presumptions.

Unlike diabetes, there's no blood test or brain scan to prove you're schizophrenic. Sure, there have been advances in theories and hypotheses, procedures that may pinpoint genes indicative of mental disorders. But principally, psychiatrists go on the words patients say, or don't say, the things they do, or don't do. And if the psychiatrist says you've got the illness, you've got it. End of.

For people like Sam, that's a real bummer. Irrespective of whether he agrees with his diagnosis or not, it's there like an amputation, with him for life. Something he must declare if he wants to learn to drive, apply for certain jobs, to travel overseas.

Why Sam, my schoolfriend Terry, and many, many others acquire the illness remains the subject for contention by people far more informed and eminent than I. Environmental factors likely play a role, like discrimination, poverty, abuse or exposure to recreational drugs; there are biological dispositions too that seem to increase susceptibility, such as a family history of the illness, foetal trauma, or comorbidities such as autism; then there are a few where there is no apparent causality, and it's just bad luck.

But why do some become unwell while others don't? I experienced difficulties growing up, saw things I shouldn't have; there are mentally unwell people in my family, and I've used my fair share of drugs. It seems unfair that I've come through relatively unscathed, while Sam hasn't.

What is unequivocal, according to the World Health Organization and Public Health England findings, is that people with schizophrenia have poorer health outcomes than the majority and will die younger than most, on average twenty years before the typical citizen. Twenty years. It's staggering.

The reasons are multifarious, as much to do with the socioeconomic outcomes, human rights violations, limited employment, health and social opportunities, and the unilaterally poor standards of living those like Sam experience. There's the long-term impact of medication and associated side-effects on physical health too, and the stigma and subjugation that comes with carrying this ball and chain.

But what's it like, learning that you have schizophrenia and living with it daily?

Before long, Sam's tells me his story, the way it really happened.

I'm in his flat now, a dusty housing association studio that carries his familiar aroma, part floral perfume, part musty sweat, plus cigarette fumes and the turpentine he soaks his paintbrushes in. Although we're in the middle of London, prime real estate for most millennials, there's something lonely about his dwellings. Apart from a single bed, a wardrobe and two camping chairs, all his belongings are crammed into cardboard boxes. Rather than family photos, the walls are furnished with sketches and paintings, all by Sam, works from over the years, documenting his decline into mental illness.

'It was during my GCSEs when it started proper. Mum and

Dad, they ran a convenience store and had big aspirations for me and my brother. I was to go to law school, and my brother to med school. They had it all mapped out. Well, my brother hit the mark, but I had other ideas. I wanted to be an artist.'

On the cusp of his A-levels, Sam grew his hair long, stopped going to mosque, started smoking a shedload of skunk, and had a secret crush on a boy he met at a Placebo gig. Photos he digs out show him as a wiry, androgenous emo-kid, much like me at his age – intense of stare, eyes dark and unrepentant.

Sam already had a lot going on in his head. The voice of his late granddad arriving at night, whispering like the sound of swishing curtains.

'It was a stressful time,' he says, lighting a roll-up. 'When Granddad was alive, he used to talk to spirits and djinn and told me ghosts were real. Even though he was dead, I could hear him. Especially after I'd been smoking. My big brother, he must've suspected something was different with me. He searched my bag, found some skunk and outed me to Mum and Dad.'

'Oh,' I say. 'How did that go down?'

'They didn't take it well.'

No shit. Sam's family ostracised him, insisting he renounce his art school dreams and attend the mosque for exorcisms. He was to cut his hair, dress decently and drop his weird friends. When he refused, they kicked him out. This was nearly a decade back, and they've never reached out to find out how he is. Sam moved to a young persons' hostel in central London. He was completely cut off.

'That's when Granddad's voice became louder,' he says. 'And mean.'

'Mean?'

'He was saying I'd brought shame on the family. I didn't deserve to be alive.'

'You believed him?'

Sam nods. 'I dropped out of college. Lost touch with my mates. I couldn't make art. When I tried, Granddad said it was worthless. Like me. All I could do was smoke.'

Indeed. Skunk became a daily go-to to plug the well of loneliness.

'What happened next?'

Sam shrugs, taps ash onto the floor. 'People began calling at my room. Strangers. I tried ignoring them. That made it worse. I'd hear them, talking about me from the hallway.'

'Who were they?'

'Spies. Operatives. Sent by my family to infiltrate my mind.'

Sam kept smoking skunk, hoping it might keep them away. On the contrary, the more he smoked, the more these visitors persisted, as stubborn as he was.

'Everything I knew, they knew. They were inside my head. I knew what I was experiencing was impossible, but that didn't make it any less real.'

Not long after, these visitors found a way into Sam's room. Seeping invisibly beneath the floorboards, whispering into his ears like his granddad had. Sam, understandably, was terrified. Then a lifeline appeared. Or so he thought.

'I met someone,' Sam says, blushing. 'A boy. He was like me. Kicked out by his family. Different. I thought he was the one. My salvation. I told him everything. He listened. I fell head over heels.'

But what could've been a tonic turned into something poisonous: Sam's crush introduced him to crystal meth and fleeced him for all his money before dumping him.

'That's when I knew,' he says.

'Knew what?'

'The boy was in on it too. I'd been used. The whole world was against me.'

Despondent and afraid, Sam began isolating, not washing, eating or drinking in case someone poisoned his food. His drug dealer, a girl in one of the neighbouring rooms, posted fresh bags of skunk through his letterbox in exchange for his dole money. For the best part of a month, he lived in darkness, the windows blacked out to prevent snipers aiming at him, the radio on to block out bugs, with no communication with the outside world.

'What happened?' I ask.

'The managers of the hostel eventually kicked the door in. They say I was huddled in a ball, hacking, blue.'

'Blue?'

'I'd swallowed a load of batteries. Granddad told me to do it.'

'Why?'

'I was heartbroken. He said it was a way to recharge my heart.'

'Jesus.'

There is a beat.

'I was brought to A&E, had surgery to remove the batteries, then got seen by the mental health team and sectioned to a hospital. For the first time, I was separated from the drugs.'

The hope was that the peculiar experiences he'd had were drug psychosis and now he was clean, they might disperse.

'But a line had been crossed,' he says.

'A line? What happened next?' I ask, intrigue now overtaking me.

'They put me onto meds,' he says. 'Antipsychotics.'

'Did they help?'

'They took the edge off what I was hearing, yeah. But the voices didn't go. Not really. I said they had in order to get out of hospital. I guess I haven't always been straight with you lot. I can still hear them now. Telling me stuff that's not real.'

'What stuff?'

'That you're against me. That I'm dirty, and don't deserve to be here.'

Don't deserve to be here. The words howl in my head.

Sam spent the next eighteen months as an inpatient on a secure adult ward: 'It was a crazy time. A year and a half, gone.'

During this admission, his initial diagnosis of psychosis was replaced with a formal one of schizophrenia. Due to his aversion to tablets and their soporific effect, he was trialled on an intramuscular depot, which led him to be referred to Alan's community mental health team, which in turn led to him meeting me.

'So there you have it,' Sam says. 'My life story.'

A strange equanimity passes between us. Like in the medication room where I impaled my hand, for a fleeting moment, the playing field is level. We're the same – two young men chatting in a flat.

'Here,' he says, 'check this out.' He reaches into his box again, handing me a scroll of butcher paper.

When I unroll it, I begin to smile. In my hands, a sketch of me stares back.

'It's not finished yet,' Sam says. 'Needs colour. A bit of refinement.'

Perhaps. But already Sam's nailed my cheekbones, thick hair, my small nose and glasses. I'm dressed how I was when I first met him, in a loose T-shirt. My expression is furtive. My right hand is wrapped in a thick bandage.

I look at Sam. His poker face has returned. Then humour sluices through and he laughs haughtily.

'Bastard,' I say, laughing with him.

Despite my concerns, I plough on through to the end of the course.

The following spring, I receive the prerequisite number of practice hours and coursework passes to gain a professional registration as a mental health nurse. Meanwhile, Alan's cancer treatment comes to an end and he makes a phased return to work. My time with his community team comes to an end too, and Sam and I say our farewells.

That summer, I begin looking for jobs. I quickly discover that mental health nurses are sought after – there are inpatient hospital jobs, prison jobs, Home Office jobs, A&E liaison jobs, private sector jobs, university jobs, charity sector jobs.

Before long, I hear about a community team specialising in mood and affective disorders, situated at the arse end of St Pancras, within the site of a former workhouse. I go to meet the manager for an informal chat. Her office walls are pasted with James Dean and Morrissey posters. Before we're past pleasantries, I'm sold.

'When can you start?' she says.

I tell her as soon as possible.

The team comprises social workers and occupational therapists, psychologists and psychiatrists, plus the nurses too. As a newly qualified staff member, I'm given a limited caseload, twenty-odd patients, nothing like the number Alan had. I get regular supervision and guidance from my manager, but even this seems a hefty quantity, for behind the diagnoses, each of these people has idiosyncrasies and quirks.

In the same way learning to drive differs from being a real-life motorist, being a qualified mental health nurse is poles apart from studying in classrooms.

I discover that many of the descriptive terms used in mental health – anhedonic, dysphoric, labile, euphoric – refer to commonplace characteristics, yet when used in this context, they can have a detrimental effect, describing symptoms, not people, pathologising thoughts, feelings, and behaviours we all experience to degrees. It's only when you meet the individual, hear their raucous laugh, see their wonky teeth, smell their sickly-sweet perfume, that you realise they are someone like you, your family member, your mate from school. Someone like Sam.

The Care Programme Approach (CPA) is the recognised framework for mental health services, in which patients with enduring and complex needs are allocated a care coordinator – in this case, me – whose job it is to oversee their treatment and support. NHS England's guidance gives examples of what this support might include help with – medication, money, housing, going out; in reality, the list is as far-reaching as the patient themselves, and their care coordinator's willingness to bend. I've known nurses who wash patients' hair, sand their floor splinters, de-grout their bathrooms. In that sense it's a holistic role. And a strange one too.

In my new role, most of my patients on CPA are experiencing significant depression, anxiety or post-traumatic stress. Some I visit at home, especially when they're too debilitated to venture out; others come to see me at the base, where we'll sit and chat about medication, their position on the psychology waiting list, their social needs, and how they're getting on.

Within a month I'm administering intramuscular injections unsupervised, liaising with chemists and GPs, applying for benefits, emergency housing, charity donations; I'm carrying out in-depth mental state examinations, referring for psychology, psychotherapy, assessments under the Mental Health Act. I help decorate flats, scrub frying pans, assemble flat packs, find plumbers, pest controllers, animal handlers, and laugh bucketloads. It's affirming, humbling, exhausting yet energising work. For chunks of the day, I don't know what I'm doing. Yet I'm glad to be doing it, nonetheless.

As I approach my first year as a qualified mental health nurse, I'm glad I stuck at it, and when I find myself in Kentish Town, passing Sam's flat, it dawns on me to drop in. This, I now know, is bad practice. Sure, we'd got on, had some banter and rapport, but Sam was my patient. To make a social call in this way blurs all kinds of boundaries.

My plan is to tell him about the job so far, hear what he's been getting up to, see some of his new artwork. Before I'm halfway to his door, I can smell the sweet, fragrant yet sickly scent of fresh cannabis smoke coming from his studio, and I hear white static noise. My insides clench. Something is wrong.

'Sam,' I say, and knock the door.

There's movement.

'Sam!' The knocks become fisted bangs.

A rattling chain and he answers through a narrow crack.

'Hey, man,' I say, relief flooding my voice.

I can see one eye, onyx black, zeroed on me. 'Who are you?' he says.

'Don't you recognise me?'

The eye carries on staring, like the telescopic sight of a rifle.

'Can I come in, Sam?' My voice is serious now.

'Why?'

'So we can talk.'

'Talk?' Another rattle of the chain, the door swings open, and there he is. 'Get in,' he says. 'Fast.'

I step into the flat and Sam quickly shuts and bolts the door. It's dark, gloomy, the windows blacked out, lightbulbs removed from fixtures; newspapers line every inch of floor and the walls have been scrawled over with felt pens declaring strange profanities – Slut. Antichrist. Sadist – all leaping out. The static is emitting from a handheld radio crunching between frequencies. The place reeks of cannabis, sweat and bad news. I breathe through my mouth to keep from gagging.

'Good to see you,' I say to Sam. 'Mind if I turn the radio off?'

He shakes his head.

'Why not?'

'They might hear us.'

'They?'

He nods. 'They're listening.'

I look at him squarely. He's wearing a dressing gown, slippers. Gone is the bandana, the edgy humour; instead, his hair is shoulder-length, matted, and he wears a thick webby beard. He seems to have shrunk, a flaccid version of the Sam I knew.

'Follow me,' he says, taking me into the flat. 'Keep your voice low.'

As soon as I enter his once-spartan living area, my heart sucks into my throat. It's in disarray – spilled ashtrays, sticky lino floors, foodstuff caked on surfaces. Bedsheets have been tacked over windows to block out light, and the wall wiring has been wrenched out from the skirting, the cables dangling like entrails. Soup and baked beans tins lie in a mountainous heap. On the kitchen surfaces are more tins, mouldy slices of bread scattered like playing cards, tubs of margarine, half-drunk bottles of Coke, a bucket containing what I assume is piss, another for God knows what. There are also two large kitchen knives glinting dully. The walls are an obscene Rorschach of archaic phrases and more obscene words.

'What . . .' I say, 'what happened?'

Sam shakes his head, reaches for an ashtray, fishes out the stub of a joint. He puts it to his lips. His fingers are caked in dirt. He digs out a lighter from the floor, fires the joint, drawing in the smoke.

'Sam! Jesus, what's going on? Why're you smoking that stuff again?'

He keeps puffing, then stubs the filter on the table. When his sleeve falls up, his forearms are laddered with self-harm cuts. Some old, most new. This is bad. I've walked into a crisis.

Working hard to keep my voice steady, I say, 'You're having a rough time?'

He nods.

'You've hurt yourself?'

Nod.

'Did no one come and check on you?'

He shakes his head.

'Let me help you, Sam.'

He taps at his brow with a yellowed fingertip, three times.

I wait for him to speak, but the tapping carries on. Then he begins to cry. Fat tears streaming down his dirty cheeks and plopping onto the rubbish-strewn floor. His eyes keep flitting from me to the two knives.

I'm flummoxed. The mental health nurse in me says to show caution; maybe call someone – the police, an ambulance. No one knows I'm here, and the door is bolted. I could be in danger.

But Jesus, this is Sam – someone I know. Not through textbooks. Not through looking at medication charts and clinical reports. But through sitting in this flat, chatting. A young man like me, trying to make sense of the world.

Before I know it, I've taken a step closer. Sam takes a

sharp intake of breath, flinches. I take another step. This time he doesn't move.

'It's OK.'

I give him a hug. It's all I can think to do.

He smells foul. His body is tremulous.

The tears keep coming.

Over the next ten minutes we talk. Making sense of Sam's narrative is hard. There are fissures in his speech. Anomalies. In mental health language, terms like 'tangential', 'derailed' or discombobulated' might be used. But these do little to conjure the strain when he enunciates, the wrenching.

From what I can gather, some kids in the area started baiting him with freebies of skunk. It'd been a few years since he last had a smoke. Sam asked for a cheeky sample. Just a small one. The skunk was good. Damn good. It fed into his creativity, improving his artwork, freeing his mind of insecurity. He started buying more from the kids, who delivered it through his letterbox in exchange for his benefits.

Now Sam didn't need to go out. It was dawning on him that his art, his mind, were uncovering a hidden masterplan. Everything was interconnected. He lay at the epicentre. His quest was to discover the truth.

But the truth never came. Instead, government spies did. Raking, punitive voices permeating the walls, trying to thwart him. Sam blacked out the windows, played his radio loud, but they found a way to seep through his porous skull tissue and into his brain. Smoking the skunk didn't help. Neither did artwork. The only way to gain a semblance of relief was through cutting his skin.

'We need to go to hospital,' I say. 'I'm calling an ambulance.'

Sam shakes his head.

'You're not well, Sam. I can't leave you.'

'I can't go back,' he sputters.

Panic rises in my throat like bile. What if he refuses to budge? I can't make him go to hospital, but I can't just leave him.

'I'll come with you,' I say.

He looks at me. 'OK,' he says.

A cab takes us to an A&E in central London. Sam's still in his dressing gown and slippers, and the driver makes a show of opening the windows and spraying down the upholstery once we exit the vehicle and enter the department.

The waiting room is rammed, toddlers bawling, builders nursing cuts, pensioners elevating legs, the displaced nodding off, nurses and health care staff doing their best to navigate through the maelstrom.

Immediately, Sam tries to turn and go, but I block his way.

'No,' I say. 'It'll be OK.'

I talk on his behalf to a churlish receptionist. At first she rolls her eyes. Then I flash my ID, say I'm a mental health nurse here with a patient in crisis. She says to take a seat and wait to be called.

'I'm scared,' Sam says.

I stay with him, staring down onlookers perturbed by his muttering, his smell, his strange attire; I stay with him when he's called up to be seen, and we go through to speak to the mental health liaison nurse, where I tell them what's happened; I stay with him as they find a private bay, tend to his cuts with steriliser and bandages; I stay as they give him something to calm him down, watching his eyelids stick together as he falls asleep. Then, finally, I feel the air seep from me in a sigh.

'Good call,' the on-call psychiatrist says, tapping his brow deferentially. 'Without you he could've been in big trouble.'

Sam's bloods show he's dehydrated and he's tested positive for cannabis – no surprises there. They decide to admit him to the general hospital for fluids and rest.

By the time I leave, it's late, past ten. I feel like I've been up for days on adrenaline and bad coffee. There's a bunch of missed calls from Clare. I call back, apologise, try my best to describe what just took place, say I'm sorry, that I love her and need a hug. She tells me that she loves me back, and I should come home for my hug now.

Sam had fallen through the cracks. Alan, his nurse, had retired post-cancer treatment. This coincided with a change in management and the introduction of a cost-cutting IT system, which meant that, somehow, Sam got overlooked.

It's a story familiar to many working in community mental health. After years of resource cuts, recruitment shortages and floundering morale, teams are treading water and the ones who suffer most are invariably our patients.

I'm angry. As I read through Sam's notes, there's a catalogue of missed opportunities. What the hell might've happened if I hadn't dropped by? He could've died in that flat. I prod his team, send a few snotty emails, voice my concern. No one replies.

A week later, I go to see Sam. By now, he's been moved to a mental health bed and placed on a section; he's been separated from the street drugs and had potent psychiatric meds pumped into him. I'd rehearsed what to say – this was a blip, he was lucky to be here and should just move on. I guess I was expecting him to be glad, for us to chat and reminisce.

When I arrive, that hope implodes. Sam's sitting up in bed, nursing a milky cup of tea. His beard is gone. He's shaved his head. He has a stark, pasty affect, like a papier mâché version of himself.

'Sam?'

He looks.

'How're you feeling?'

He keeps looking.

'Sam?'

'Go,' he whispers.

'Sam, what's–'

'I said go. I don't want to see you again.'

I say something else, and he tells me to fuck off. It goes on this way until I finally step back just in time to miss the cup of tea hurled at me that splatters over the wall.

'Maybe it's because you care,' the nurse in charge of Sam's care says as I describe this rebuttal. 'He's not used to it. It hurts.'

'Why?'

'Because he knows you'll eventually leave him.'

It makes sense, but that doesn't make it easier.

'So what should I do?'

'Nothing.'

'Nothing?'

'You've done your best.'

She's right, of course. I had done my best. It was starting

to dawn on me that the hefty textbooks and fancy psychiatric words would only take me so far. This job is about you and me, sharing our humanity, learning how little we know about who we are, and how alike that makes us.

A few months after that visit to the hospital, where I'd narrowly dodged Sam's tea, a parcel arrives for me at the office, sent by Royal Mail special delivery. There's my name printed in a heavy pastel scrawl. Before opening it, I know what's inside.

I unravel the butcher paper portrait and smile. It's the finished pastel sketch showing me as a trainee. There's no notes or messages, just Sam's signature in the bottom right corner. Carefully, I pin the sketch above my desk and stare at it, feeling a strange warmth that hadn't been there a moment ago.

I've had other jobs since and have no idea how Sam's currently doing. It wouldn't surprise me to learn that he'd hit the big time with his art, secured commissions, been the success I knew he had it in him to be. Likewise, it wouldn't surprise me if something terrible had happened. To survive mental health care, you must accept the *not* knowing.

But I do know that in a dusty office in a central London community mental health team, that portrait of me signed by Sam still hangs on a wall. The likeness is good, albeit a version of me from years back, but if there was any doubting who it is, I can be identified by the furtive expression on my face, and the bandage around my impaled hand.

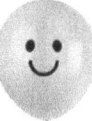

Maladjusted

ACCORDING TO COLIN, the patient stood to my left, of all the public toilets in Camden Town, the one we are presently standing in is the mankiest.

It's Tuesday morning, a dazzling, late-summer day in London. Shoppers, tourists, commuters intersect above us, trampling the streets like wildebeest. But down here, in this underground Gents, we're interned in the intestines of the city, a septic tank of gloom.

A caged light flickers limply, drawing out the shadows rather than illuminating the space. Walls are cracked Victorian tiles, snot green; floors a sticky terracotta ceramic smeared in grime. It's eerily quiet, just an echoey drip-drip from cisterns and the thud of machines and motor vehicles. Left are the urinals clogged with rivers of piss, cigarette butts floating downstream like canoes. Right are the cubicles, eight in total, two with doors ripped off, showing an eruption of soiled bog roll and human waste that contributes to the smell.

Ah, the smell. I try to breathe through my mouth, but

several times a half-sniff slips through. It's warm, foul, a putrid hit attacking my olfactory senses with a sledgehammer, tugging at me to go. But go I cannot. I'm here for professional reasons. This is about Colin. This is Colin's treatment.

He's wearing All Stars, jeans, a plain T-shirt. Although he's in his late twenties, he could pass as a nineteen-year-old, with his wispy stubble, creamy skin and a neat preppy side-parting. Right now, his eyes are closed. Hands loose by his sides. He's breathing deeply, diaphragmatically. In through the nose. Out from the mouth. A fugue. This is the third toilet we've stood in this morning. Colin knows all the public conveniences in the borough intimately, ranking them in order of disgust.

This is odd. Very odd. But being a mental health nurse, as I've been for two years now, means being exposed to life's oddities on a regular basis. Right now I could be drinking a frappé latte, strolling across the heath, rooting through record shops. Instead, I'm a grown man stood beside another grown man in a public toilet and–

''Scuse me.'

Colin starts, as do I.

Behind us, a flat-capped elderly gent wants to get past. We step aside. As he walks between us, he brushes shoulders with Colin. Like a marionette pulled taut, Colin's body tenses.

'Easy,' I say.

The old man bales.

Colin scrubs the spot where contact was made as if the skin were infected. A vein pulses in his neck. The man stands by the urinal, unzips, looks at us again. The light tinkle of water spraying on the cisterns. Mid-flow, he lets out a trump.

'I think I'm ready to go,' Colin says.

Restraining myself from whooping, I say, 'You're sure? We can stay a bit longer if you need to.'

'I'm sure,' Colin says. 'It's been helpful.'

The old man hawks, spits. Then he zips up, walks towards us, no intention of washing his hands. His stare is like an ice burn.

'Don't mind me asking, boys,' he says, 'what the heck are you doing?'

I've known Colin for three months now. Three strained yet strangely rewarding months. I was allocated to work with him following his discharge from a specialist inpatient unit in south London where they treat the severest cases of obsessive-compulsive disorder.

OCD is one of the most misunderstood mental disorders. How many times have you heard people drop the term into conversation, adjectivising it, saying someone's being 'a bit OCD', or 'that's a bit OCD-ey' in reference to vaguely ritualistic or repetitive behaviours with an air of comedy and daftness to them.

In fact, OCD is a debilitating, remarkably *un*funny condition, what the World Health Organization determines as being in the top ten disabling illnesses, affecting loss of income and quality of life. As its name would imply, OCD is a conflation of obsessions and compulsions that are insidiously linked, unique to the individual and never pleasurable or enjoyable. Being passionate about football, shopping, sex, or stamp, autograph or book collecting are far cries from OCD, which is characterised by shame and misery, grim repetition of the same acts again and again, any choice to abstain removed.

In many ways, OCD manifests like an addiction. Treatment will depend on the individual, the severity of symptoms, the impact on a person's livelihood, their social support network and their readiness to address the problem. For some, group or individual therapy might be sufficient; for others, a combination of intensive therapy and psychotropic medication is necessary; for a few, an intensive inpatient period of treatment is deemed proportionate.

Whatever the support, National Institute for Health and Care Excellence (NICE) guidelines are clear that towards the end of treatment, health care professionals should help sufferers practise the principles learned to manage symptoms if they return. It parallels the alcoholic who must maintain a programme of recovery to keep their sobriety: an OCD sufferer must keep up a regimented scheme for the obsessions and compulsions to remain at bay. It is this that has prompted my input with Colin, and which led us into this murky public loo.

Prior to his admission, Colin's life had been stricken. His obsessions orbited around hygiene, cleanliness, avoidance of dirt, grub, bacteria. In response, his compulsions were ever-increasing measures to manage these preoccupations – cleaning, bleaching, scrubbing again and again, all to temper the belligerent monster in his head.

I first went to see him when he was poised for discharge from the aforementioned unit. He'd been there for a month, during which time he'd made massive improvements. He was happy to talk, sitting on his neatly made bed. The way I remember it, our first encounter went like this:

'I knew what I was doing, how I was living, was wrong. Washing my hands or brushing my teeth would take half an hour. Sometimes I'd scrub so much I'd draw blood. From the moment I got up, all I could think about was cleaning and germs and bacteria and ways to get rid of them. It wasn't that I was blinkered; I knew I was ill. But that realisation wasn't enough to stop it. I hoped that if I carried on, something would change. *I'd* change. Instead, I kept on cleaning. More and more. Going insane. Isn't there a saying about that?'

I nod. 'Insanity's doing the same thing and expecting different results?'

Colin smiles. 'Believe it or not, when I was young, I was a messy kid. Always muddy and grubby. My bedroom was a right tip. Then, when I was six, Mum died of sepsis, and it was just me and Dad. I became tidy. I liked things to be ordered. I used to look for patterns. Symmetry. I'd tap walls and tables and make special rhythms. I'd check I'd locked doors like ten times before going out. Walking on cracks in paving stones was bad luck. I had these chants I'd repeat every night – if I didn't do all these things, bad stuff would happen, like it did to Mum, and it would be my fault. It felt like there was this secret thing I was carrying around, an invisible ball and chain that was getting heavier and heavier. It lasted till secondary school.'

'What changed?' I ask.

'Dad just said to me, "Son, you need to sort yourself out." And it just fell away, all by itself. It stayed that way for years.'

During which time Colin headed to university, got a good job as a software manager with a city tech firm, met a girl, and they moved in together. Life was good. But when he reached his mid-twenties, things changed again. First, the girl left him for someone else. Austerity hit, and he lost the job. Then his dad had a stroke that left him in ICU. Within weeks he developed a chest infection and died. Colin was alone.

'I moved into Dad's old flat. The place was dusty and grim. The bed where he died was as he left it. Everything was a reminder of him.

'Suddenly, I got it in my head that maybe he got sick because of the dirt at home. Maybe Mum did too, all those years ago. Maybe that was why I'd lost my job and my girlfriend. Because of bacteria. I know it sounds nuts, but I couldn't shake the idea. And so I developed this interest in keeping things clean. Very clean.'

Correct. Colin went to ever-increasing lengths to dampen these thoughts. Hours were spent on hand and knee, bleaching floors, sanitising the shower, scraping the oven for crumbs of charred food. Washing his body was a convoluted process, beginning at his feet, slowly working up his whole body. If a mistake was made, no matter how small, he had to start the whole process again.

Shopping was delivered through online delivery, always deposited on the doorstep late at night so that Colin could retrieve the goods under the cover of darkness when there were fewer people and less chance of infection. Once the purchases were inside the flat, he would begin the complex process of cleaning the cans and containers, wiping them down with antibacterial spray, checking them meticulously. Otherwise something terrible would happen. And it would all be his fault.

'I was a prisoner,' Colin says. 'A prisoner of *me*.'

At the time of his admission, he couldn't leave the flat unless he was wearing a boilersuit, complete with oxygen mask and gas cylinders. Neighbours would stare at this strange astronaut figure.

This went on for five years, and it might've continued longer. It was only when Colin was gripped with an agonising toothache that he was forced to take the drastic measure of visiting the dentist. Donned in his boilersuit, he entered the local practice and pleaded to be seen.

The receptionist would've been within her rights to call the police at the sight of this bizarre person. But by providence she had a family member diagnosed with OCD. While Colin was having an infected molar extracted, she printed off some pamphlets and numbers for an OCD support line that she gave him as he rushed out.

'Till then,' he says, 'I'd never heard of this illness.'

Colin self-referred for a course of cognitive behavioural therapy, the first-line evidence-based treatment for his condition. The prospect of navigating through the filthy streets of London for therapy was impossible, so it was delivered online. Over six sessions, a therapist broke down Colin's thoughts, feelings, behaviours and bodily sensations in a hot-cross bun diagram, showing how they were interlinked. His pathological thinking errors were compelling him to feel and act in these bizarre ways that were ruining his quality of life.

'What the therapist said made perfect sense,' Colin explains. 'But when she asked me to do stuff about it and challenge myself, I couldn't. That made me feel a bigger failure. And the cleaning ramped up even more.'

Next, he was trialled on a course of antidepressants, selective serotonin reuptake inhibitors (SSRIs), which he had delivered from the chemist shop to his doorstep in blister packs. These had some benefits.

'They made me sleep, which helped. But that was all. And before long I was on the max dose, and still stuck with me inside my head.'

Colin's therapist admitted that he had run out of ideas.

'That's when things got bad.'

'How bad?' I ask.

He looks at his hands. Small, neat hands that he'd tried to end his life with, tying a cord around his neck, attempting to hang himself in the kitchen.

'I couldn't even get that right, though.'

'What do you mean?' I ask.

'I tied the rope to a light fixture in the ceiling, stood on a chair and leapt off. Instead of killing me, I brought the light out of the plasterwork and ended up in a heap on the floor. Dust went everywhere. The kitchen was a tip.'

'Wow,' I say. 'You're lucky.'

Colin shrugs. 'You know what my first thought was? Not that I could've died, but that I'd made a God-awful mess and would need to tidy it all up pronto to keep the germs away.'

Despite the sombre tone, we both laugh.

Shortly afterwards, Colin's therapist referred him to specialist mental health services and my team, and, once the severe extent of his illness was ascertained, a decision was made to seek inpatient care, which Colin embarked on, knowing that his life depended on it.

The treatment was tough, designed to combat the

obsessions that had become so engrained. Exposure therapy is easy to explain, hard to do. After identifying the route of the obsessions – in Colin's case, a need for cleanliness – he was to counter these by exposing himself to *un*cleanliness, a counteraction.

'It started low level: twenty minutes of hand washing rather than thirty; allowing for a few specks of grub on the carpet to remain. Pretty quickly, though, they ramped it up.

'Leaving the toilet seat unclean after urinating. Shaking hands with strangers. Showering only once a day. Realising that bad things wouldn't happen.'

The next step was immersing himself in and around filthy environments, the stinkier and nastier the better, public conveniences being the obvious choice. It isn't some fetish, or a way of indulging scatological interests: it's maintenance work.

'So how are you finding it?' I ask him a short while after leaving the public toilet in Camden Town. We're in a greasy spoon off the high street, both nursing a coffee. Normally, the reek of refried oil and cooked meat would turn my guts; now, compared to where we've been, it's sublime.

'There's good days and bad days,' Colin says. 'Sometimes I feel like I'm on top of it. Then suddenly the thoughts grab me by the throat.' He wraps his hand around his jugular, where the light indents from when he tried to hang himself are still visible. 'Today feels like that, a little.'

With Colin the stakes are high and as his care coordinator, I can sense he's holding back. 'What's up?' I say.

He flicks his fringe out of his eyes.

'Colin, you can talk to me.'

His pale cheeks blush. 'I've met someone,' he says. 'A girl.'

'Oh,' I say. 'That's good. Right?'

'Kind of,' he says. 'I mean, she's nice. She goes to one of my support groups. She's got OCD too. It means I don't have to explain everything, which is handy.'

'What's she like?'

'With her, the obsessions and compulsions came out as hoarding. Apparently, the environmental health had to declutter her flat due to the fire risk. Books and magazines sky-high. She was sleeping in the hallway because she couldn't get into any of the rooms. After they'd taken everything it took her two weeks to hit all the charity shops and free newspaper drop-offs across town and pack every room again. Poor thing's worse than me.'

'She sounds a real catch,' I say.

We laugh, and then the laughter fades and we look at our coffees. Colin, I've noticed, has arranged his cup, saucer and spoon equidistantly apart on the table. Before touching the handle of his cup, he gives it a small rub with a serviette.

'It's coming back,' he says. 'I can feel it. Last night, I started cleaning. Nothing like before. Just some dusting. A bit of polishing. But I felt dirty after. The flat, me, it all felt dirty. Maybe I'm not ready for this.'

I pause, carefully selecting my words. 'Getting into a new relationship is tough. Brings out all kinds of anxieties.'

He nods.

'But if you don't take a few risks, you'll never find out what you're capable of.'

Another nod.

'Apart from having OCD, what else is this lady like?'

For the first time, Colin smiles broadly. 'She's cute.'

Over the next ten minutes, Colin tells me about his new acquaintance, her quirks, her interests. His face is clenched with emotion, but I know he wants this, and tell him as much.

'It'll be OK,' I say. 'You've got the tools to stay on top of this thing. Right?'

'Right,' Colin says.

My coffee is cold. I push it aside. 'I better go. What are you up to?'

Colin smiles thinly, and his cheeks blanch red. Despite the heat, an icy finger runs up my spine.

'There's another toilet a few minutes up the road. Place is a real state. Right now, I think I need it. Have you got time?'

I feel a sinking inside, coupled with a Pavlovian reflux taste of bile. Every instinct screams to lie, make something up, tell him I need to scoot off to my next appointment rather than stand in another cacky public Gents. But I can't do that. Colin needs this. If I bullshit him, I'd be abusing our relationship.

'Ten minutes,' I say.

He grins. 'You sure?'

'I'm sure.'

'It's a weird job you do, isn't it?'

I tell him it is.

I skip lunch, the toilet fumes quelling my appetite, and head back to the team base to percolate a second coffee and write some notes.

Our base office is a 1970s structure that screams public

sector: the exterior is brown brickwork and grey cladding, the interior anaemic wood laminate and bleary strip lights. Posters for mental health support groups are crinkling from the wall and an administrator sits behind a desk tapping a keyboard with the enthusiasm of a prisoner on execution day. To an outsider it would appear a wholly grim place to work. Yet there is a strange camaraderie here and a lack of airs and graces among staff. On my first day I passed what I assumed was a patient stood outside the building chuffing on a roll-up, muttering incoherently. Ten minutes later said patient wandered into the office and introduced himself as a social worker. Straightaway, I knew we'd get on.

The senior medics and lead psychologists are granted their own private offices. The rest of us hot-desk in a cramped, open-plan room, scrambling for a corner of table from where to log on. Today I'm sharing the space with the aforementioned social worker, Glynn, who is attacking his keyboard with his index fingers; there's a keen young assistant psychologist here too, Emily, touch-typing with one hand, flicking through hand-scribed notes with the other; there's a seventy-one-year-old mental health nurse, Gladys, trying to figure out how to reset her laptop password after being booted out of our Trust's prehistoric IT system; and there's me.

Quickly, I bang out some notes about my meeting with Colin. Mental health nurses must be adept at carrying out mental state examinations, MSEs for short, in which key areas about a patient's presentation are considered. A typical MSE would cover appearance, behaviour, speech, mood, affect, thought, perceptions, cognitions. In addition, there will be the mandatory questions about sleep, diet, side-effects from meds, a measurement of capacity and insight, and thoughts to hurt or kill self or others.

With Colin's notes done, I scan through my caseload, seeing if anything untoward has happened to anyone since I last looked. I care coordinate thirty-one patients, all as complex as Colin, all requiring a mental health professional to oversee their community support. Thirty-one is a lot, but nothing compared to some colleagues: sometimes it feels I'm on top of it, other times as if I'm just about treading water.

As with most community mental health teams, ours is short-staffed, and recruitment of substantive posts is a challenge. To fill holes, Trusts either haemorrhage money on locums or accept gaping holes and associated risks. Despite the government's pledge to deliver thousands more into the mental health workforce, the vacancies remain, and with the abolition of nurses' bursaries and the introduction of student fees, the lures are even less apparent and the future looks bleak.

I'd planned to use the next couple of hours to catch up on admin, revise support plans, risk assessments, applying to a furniture charity for a patient who's just moved into a flat, appealing a disability benefit rejection for another. Before I can, an email has flashed on my screen. It's from Martin, husband of Dulcie, another of my patients. It reads: 'D's not doing well today. Needs her fix, but I can't rouse her. Any chance you can help?'

I sigh. My plans will need to change.

I type back to Martin that I'm on my way, grab my bag and scoot out, leaving my second coffee of the day undrunk.

*

Anyone who claims that mental illness is an equal opportunities affliction needs to be put right. If you're socioeconomically deprived and experience the housing problems, cost of living crises, employment difficulties, educational challenges – and the breadth of other disadvantages that are synonymous with poverty – you're more likely to suffer mental health problems too. The writing's on the wall.

But I'd challenge the notion that one person's suffering is more justified than another's because of how much or little they possess. I've met hedge fund bankers in the pits of depression, aristocratic ladies crippled by anxiety. Pain is pain. No one has the monopoly on it.

With Dulcie, the turmoil she experiences is scorched further because of the guilt she feels over her wealth, that she believes makes her undeserving of mental illness. Her main dwelling (she has several homes) is one of those gated mansions situated on tree-lined streets in northwest London. Her neighbours are footballers, Russian oligarchs and Persian princes. Visitors are cleaners, interior designers, security guards, chauffeurs – not mental health nurses.

I've visited several times and have grown familiar with the lengthy security gate entrance, the probing stares from the guard at the door. The interior is as plush and pristine as any interior on *Grand Designs*. Curtains are silk chiffon, chandeliers shiny crystal, the parquet floors buffed to the highest sheen. Surrounding me are objets d'art – opulent ceramics and asymmetric sculptures I suspect are worth more than my annual income.

At the foot of the first flight of stairs stands Martin. A former executive with one of the oil giants, there are still signs of the corporate man in him – his Italian loafers, creaseless chinos, Ralph Lauren polo shirt, silver-fox hair brushed back – but there's a stoop to his shoulders, bags beneath his eyes. He should've been enjoying his retirement, yachting in the Bahamas, but the last ten years have been blighted by Dulcie's bouts of depression.

'Thanks for coming,' he says, offering a handshake.

'No problem,' I say. 'What's been going on?'

'Another bad night. I don't think I can get her to hospital by myself.' He sniffs; for an awful second I'm sure he can smell debris from my toilet visit with Colin. Then his eyes fill and I realise it's coming from somewhere else. 'Let's go up and see her.'

For some, depressive illness comes as a reaction to life circumstances. For others, there's an organic cause, some imbalance in the neurotransmitters associated with mood. Dulcie's disorder is an unhappy fusion of both.

Despite years of attempts to conceive, and thousands spent on fertility treatment, her and Martin's dream to have a baby failed to materialise. When the perimenopause came early, the harsh truth that a baby would never appear slammed home. This realisation, conflated with the hormonal changes her body was going through, was enough to send this once-buoyant business consultant into the greyest of lows.

Dulcie is in her bedroom, the lights off, curtains drawn. As my eyes adjust, I take her in. Depression doesn't only affect the mind of the patient. The physical impact can be profound. She's in bed, a blanket drawn to her chin, the shrunken body of a child outlined beneath. Her face is oatmeal grey. Her hair is matted, a hoary web of salty black, and her lips are dry and pinched shut.

There was a time when I'd have romanticised depression, envisioning it as the natural state for those with a disposition for melancholia, like me. In truth, at its most acute depression is a debilitating state that strips the sufferer of hope, and often those around them too. Gillian Flynn's protagonist in *Sharp Objects* stated so eloquently: 'They always call (it) the blues . . . but to me, it's urine yellow, washed out, exhausted miles of weak piss.'

It's a tough illness, and tough to be around, sucking the marrow from life, closing doors, dimming lights, leaving a feeling of impotence and failure.

But Dulcie's depression can improve. The fix Martin referred to in his email is electroconvulsive therapy, that maligned *One Flew Over the Cuckoo's Nest* treatment that I've subsequently seen to be an elixir for certain patients.

The science behind ECT is unclear. A psychiatrist I knew once described its process as being akin to a snowstorm jug shaken up, the careening flakes like the neurotransmitters sparked to life by the electric current passed through the cranium. Undoubtedly a blunt tool that carries certain risks, it is generally given to patients for whom other options, such as medication and talking therapy, have been explored first.

Like so many treatments in mental health care, ECT was discovered by chance. In the early twentieth century, an Italian neuropsychiatrist was researching epilepsy using electric shocks to induce convulsions. When it was found that the results impacted on mood and affect, a new form of convulsive treatment was trialled for mental patients. The results proved astonishing. Visit the Science Museum in London and you can see a rudimentary machine that was used in the mid-century, the two probes that deliver the shock resembling the headphones of a 1980s Walkman.

For some, a course of ECT is prescribed while the patient is admitted to hospital; others, like Dulcie, will be administered 'top-up' ECT to block a relapse. The treatment is painless, delivered under general anaesthetic. There are, however, side-effects – short-term memory loss being the most common. But having seen the debilitating effects depression can have, I would argue this to be an acceptable sacrifice. And for Dulcie, it's essential.

I make a few calls from the hallway, inform her consultant of the situation and that I'll be accompanying her to the hospital. Then I say to Martin, 'Come on. Let's help her up.'

We approach on opposite sides of the bed. Dulcie's flat eyes gaze up at us like two black washers. Carefully, Martin pulls the sheets back. Dulcie resists, but her grip is weak. When he prises her fingers away, there's no fight.

We take her under each armpit and then lift her to a seated position. She's wearing a silk nightie and slippers and feels like a bag of bones. I can tell Martin has sprayed her with perfume earlier, something expensive, but even this can't mask the sour tang of urine from her body, nor the stale must from her breath. Slowly, we negotiate her from the bed. Her feet barely touch the floor. We shuffle with her towards the door, downstairs and to the car outside.

The three of us – Martin, Dulcie and I – sit together in the back while the driver glides his Chrysler through midday traffic in the direction of the hospital. Despite the warm weather, Dulcie has a blanket around her. She remains mute, staring flatly as we glide through the streets of central London traffic. Outside there is music, food smells, bustle, the heat mirage caused by static and exhaust making the air seem to shudder. It jars with the interior of the car, where the energy seems depleted, the colours diluted.

'Not long now, love,' Martin says, squeezing her hand.

When we arrive at the hospital, we help Dulcie out, one on each side.

'Where are you taking me?' she mutters as we approach the reception, her voice little more than a husk.

'For your treatment,' Martin says.

She goes stiff. For a moment I fear she might collapse, or even try to flee. Dulcie's depression wants her to stay ill. But something else – a will to live – keeps her going.

Through double doors, more double doors, a lift upstairs, and within minutes we're in a small clinical space that to an onlooker could be mistaken for a dentist's room. Centre stage is a reclining chair with electro-motor adjustments to make the user vertical or horizontal. Behind, there's a small square electric device with wires and cables attached, along with a pair of paddle-shaped plates. Two men are here – both wearing suits. One is a consultant anaesthetist, the other a psychiatrist. There's also an ECT charge nurse with specialist training. They are all unshocked at Dulcie's condition. Patients referred for ECT are often dangerously ill.

Martin helps her forward and she perches on the seat, and then lies down. The psychiatrist looks at her and smiles. What follows is a series of routine questions to Dulcie and Martin about Dulcie's mood, physical health, obvious triggers for this decline.

'She started to feel poorly over the weekend,' Martin said. 'I was hoping it was a blip. Then, three days back, she took to bed. And she hasn't got up.'

'Not missed any of her meds?' the psychiatrist asks.

Martin shakes his head.

'And you're still seeing the therapist?'

'Twice a week,' Martin says. 'Before this happened.'

While they speak, the anaesthetist starts drawing up solutions into large syringes, then applying latex gloves. Meanwhile, the nurse checks dials on the machine, lifting the paddles, examining them.

'Well,' the psychiatrist says, 'let's see what we can do to improve things.'

The anaesthetist rolls up Dulcie's sleeve, examines her forearm for a viable vein. The skin is loose, peppered with indents from previous treatments, the venous access compromised by her poor fluid intake. He wraps a tourniquet around her bicep. With an artist's precision he slips a canular needle in. Dulcie doesn't flinch.

'Ready?' the psychiatrist says, looking at the nurse, who's prepped all the apparatus, and nods.

Dulcie grunts something. 'You're OK, love,' Martin says, and brushes back her hair.

When the anaesthetic goes in, she closes her eyes, and they stay closed. There is no change to her expression at all; no loosening of the jowls, just a stretching of her breathing. Her stats appear on a monitor – pulse, blood pressure, oxygen saturation. After a moment, the anaesthetist inserts a protective guard into her mouth.

'I think we're ready,' the psychiatrist says.

I stand with Martin by the door; we are like two sentries.

Administering ECT is a procedure that only a trained psychiatrist can do. He lifts the two paddles in each hand and then places them against Dulcie's upper temple, one left, one right, parallel to each other. He looks at the nurse, nods. The nurse flicks a switch.

The shock is silent. Dulcie's body recoils. Her spine rises. Her nostrils flare. The stats on the machine go berserk. Martin stands rigid. Heat pulses from him. His hands splay on the door frame.

Dulcie starts fitting, sharp, gyratory movements. Tendons rise to the surface of her skin. She bites down on the mouth guard, her back arching. The two doctors and nurse are unperturbed. They check the monitors, which begin to steady, and Dulcie steadies too, her jerks and pulses calming, her spine coming down, until she is gradually at rest.

'Look,' Martin says to me. 'She's coming back.'

It's barely minutes since the shock was administered. The anaesthetic is wearing off. Dulcie's eyes have opened. Something is awoken in her mind. It's slight, but irrefutable.

I've witnessed ECT a few times. The wonder at the sight of this intimate, undignified, yet restorative treatment has never lessened.

The nurse and Martin help Dulcie up, offer a sweetened cup of tea. Her hair is frizzed up. When she speaks, the words are shaky and slurred, but there's a vibrancy that wasn't there before.

'There's too much sugar in this,' she says, holding up the Styrofoam cup of tea to Martin.

'It's how you normally like it, love,' he says. 'After–'

'After getting zapped through the head like Frankenstein's monster and brought back to life?'

Martin clears his throat. The ECT nurse looks at me, grinning.

'What now?' Dulcie says.

Martin smiles. His eyes are wet.

'For heaven's sake, what's the matter, you daft bear?'

He puts a hand to his mouth and says, 'How about we go home?'

By the time I've seen Dulcie and Martin back to their house, it's gone five. I'm flagging from the heat, travel, and all the fraught emotions. I've been working since eight, no break, no let-ups. That evening, I'm meant to be going out with Clare, now my wife, to see some art-house film in town. Really, I should be heading back to our flat to freshen up.

But mental health staff often go the extra mile and there's a final visit of the day I can't swerve. Of all the patients on my caseload, Harry is perhaps the saddest, and the most frustrating. I've been unable to make a dent in his armour. And today, it's time to acknowledge that.

Harry lives in a looming council block, up on the seventeenth floor. Whenever I visit, I stop to admire the expansive view of London. Beneath the shimmering clouds poke the stems of buildings – St Paul's, the Shard, Big Ben – eternals of this city.

For many, a view like this would be reason to venture out. But Harry hasn't seen this view, the city, or even been outside the confines of his home's interior for over two decades. He wants to, but something gets in the way.

'Hi, Harry,' I say, sitting opposite him in his lounge.

He nods and smiles unhappily.

Harry is slumped in his late dad's armchair. A big, flaccid man, he fills it like a foot in a broken-in boot. He's grown heavy and weak from years of over-feeding and inactivity, and is now obese. His greasy dark hair is choppy from homemade cuts, his teeth yellowing, his skin a clammy, febrile grey. He wears a vest, shorts and sliders from which his large feet swell. His face is jowly and inert, everything seeming to sag – everything apart from his eyes. They are beady and trusting, the eyes of a sad mongrel.

'So,' I say. 'How've you been?'

Instead of answering, he turns towards his mum, Eileen, perched on a chair at the small Formica dining table opposite. A fiery, pint-sized woman somewhere in her mid-seventies, she's dressed in a moth-eaten jumper, baggy men's jeans and Dunlop trainers. Her hair is grey, her shoulders, elbows, knuckles jut out like clothes hangers, and her expression is clenched with emotion, like an arthritic fist.

'He's been having a tough time,' she says. 'It's because you're abandoning him.' She pulls a deck of Sovereigns out and lights one, tapping ash into a tray between tubs of red and brown sauce. Within seconds, the lounge is a fug of smoke.

'I'm not abandoning him,' I say. 'I just don't know if there's more I can do.'

'Sorry,' Harry says to me. 'I've wasted your time, haven't I?'

'Don't be daft,' I say. 'Now just wasn't the right time for us to work together.'

'Hm,' Eileen says.

MALADJUSTED

I look at her. Her lower lip trembles. Hot tears rivulet down her cheeks. She seems unaware.

Earlier, she'd greeted me at the door with her usual mix of deference and sarcasm: 'Hello, Mister Nurse. He's been lookin' forward to seeing you.' He being Harry. Everything Eileen says comes through the lens of her son.

Harry was just five when his dad, her husband, died from a sudden heart attack. Described by Eileen as a shy, heavyset boy, Harry was bullied at school because of his weight and clinginess to his mum. When said bullies cornered him, beat him, scared him so much he began to wet his pants at the thought of going to school, Eileen made the decision to remove him from mainstream education and help him regain his confidence.

Her efforts at home-schooling bellyflopped. Harry became a homebody, fearing the outside and eventually refusing to venture anywhere. While his peers were reaching adolescence, hitting milestones, his life shrivelled like a grape in the sun.

Rather than challenge this, Eileen let him stay home. Having her son with her meant she wasn't as lonely as before. She brought him food, clothes, tended to him. She enabled his decline – a mistake, she now knows, for it allowed this strange, symbiotic relationship to forge between them in the decades that followed.

The referral to my community mental health team came from Eileen. Deep down, she knows the sand is running through the hourglass and she needs to get support for her son now. For Eileen has a secret she hasn't told Harry: a lump, discovered on her right breast, is growing.

That support arrived in me. A mental health nurse whose

remit was to encourage Harry – whose official diagnoses are chronic agoraphobia, social anxiety and post-traumatic stress – out of his slumber and into the real world. When I began, I knew it wouldn't be easy. Harry's been stuck for a long time. In every town and city there are people like him. Reclused. Housebound. Struggling out of sight.

In the past few months, he's been prescribed a combination of antidepressants – Mirtazapine and Venlafaxine, colloquialised to California Rocket Fuel when taken together due to their 'firing up' effect. I've done my best to use motivational interviewing, behavioural activation, to challenge his catastrophic thinking and coax him out. I've now come to accept that it isn't working. Harry isn't even pre-contemplative about tackling his illnesses. The one time I got him out his front door, he vomited with anxiety. It's time to step back.

I look around the small two-bedder he and Eileen share, aware that this will be my last visit to this sad, familiar space. No flat-screen TVs, smartphones, laptops. The telly is a 1970s Sony machine wired up to a Betamax cassette recorder. The shelves have a collection of tapes, the titles written in neat felt pen – *Back to the Future*; *The Lost Boys*; *Teen Wolf*; *St Elmo's Fire*. There are more posters tacked up from that era – Bridget Fonda, Patricia Arquette, *Flashdance*. It's as if time has frozen in this flat. And in a way, it has.

'Sorry,' Harry repeats, his voice a puffy, cockney wheeze, like a character from a Dickens novel. 'It's nice to see you.'

He means this. Apart from Eileen, I'm the only person he ever sees. He spends his days watching his dad's videos, reading his books, sitting in his armchair and staring.

'He thinks you're giving up on him,' Eileen says.

I look at her. 'I'm not,' I say.

'He wants to get better,' she says, her voice cracking. 'Don't you, boy? Tell him.'

Harry nods obediently.

'Isn't there no more you can do?'

I sigh. Over the past few months, there's been a lot of sighing in this flat.

'Will you still come back,' Harry eventually asks, 'after work, now and then? We can watch a video together. Chat.'

I smile, and I shake my head. 'That's not how it works. But when you're ready–' I look at Eileen, 'when you're *both* ready, it's easy to get back in touch with the team. We can pick up where we left off.'

Eileen's lip trembles. I know what she's thinking. How much time does she have?

I shake both their hands – Harry's large and clammy, Eileen's small and brittle.

Leaving, I know in my heart that Harry and Eileen's situation is unsustainable. If her lump doesn't get her, something else will, and when that happens Harry's life will be devastated. I can't imagine how he will cope. There's no one to look out for him. Maybe it will be his making. Or maybe his end. But right now, neither is ready or capable of changing. It's an impasse.

Out on the balcony, as I await the lift, Eileen comes out. I brace myself for an earful. Instead, she hesitates, hands clenching and unclenching, and she gives me a hug. She smells of must, and age, and desperation.

*

That evening, Clare and I just about make the film at the Curzon, a French drama with subtitles and lots of morose stares. It got good reviews, but I take little in. My mind pulses with the day's events: the things I did, didn't do, the words I said, and those that I didn't.

After, we go for pizza. Clare knows I'm elsewhere but doesn't ask why, which I appreciate. A social science researcher and fitness instructor, her work is oceans away from mine. To try to explain the quiet intimacies, the peculiarities, the nuances of a day like today is hard, even with her. Instead, we discuss the film, order pudding, talk about the future. We make tentative plans to go away that Christmas, and maybe redecorate our dinky flat come the new year. Life is good.

In my heart, though, I know something is about to change.

Cemetery Gates

MARY RETURNS HER cup of tea to the table.

We are in the sitting room of her terraced house, where she lives alone. It's daytime, mid-afternoon, yet the blinds are drawn, the lights off. She's wearing slippers and a dressing gown. Dust motes hover in the static air.

'Sorry,' she says. 'I'm not much company today.'

'You've nothing to apologise for,' I say.

'Eventually I'll get back on my feet.'

Perhaps. But Mary's got a long way to go. In the months I've known her, we've tried many things to help her reconnect with the woman she was, including digging out trinkets and photos from before, a psychological way to trigger hope, activate memories, wrench her from this slump. Those photos show Mary beaming, her hair vibrant blonde, not tired brown like it is now, her eyes warm, seeking, not these grey, heavy things.

'Have you been sleeping?'

She shrugs.

'Eating?'

Shrug.

'Have you been getting out at all?'

Rather than answer, Mary purses her lips. Then she looks above the mantle: a framed school portrait rests there, showing a mousy-haired teenage boy with sharp blue eyes.

'He'd have been about your age now.'

I nod.

'You think about him much? Those chats you had?'

'Sometimes,' I say.

'He liked you.'

'Yes,' I say. 'I liked him.'

When I was first asked to work with Mary, the surname chimed but I didn't clock why. Then, when I met her, a stone in my memory dislodged. But not fully. It was only when I saw the photo above the mantle, really studied the teenage boy's face, that I got it. All at once I fell back through time and landed in that strange, crushing day when the first patient I'd cared for took his life.

Mary is Jack's mother. Jack being the young man from the ward who put himself on the train tracks when I was a trainee. The years since his death have been cruel to her. In the aftermath, her career as a secondary maths teacher was the first hit, her grief rendering her incapable of performing like before; her marriage to Jack's dad followed, him blaming her, her blaming him, neither knowing how to make sense of their only child's senseless departure.

Now her life has wilted. In her mid-fifties, she looks like she's in her seventies. She rarely goes out, speaks to anyone.

She exists in this suet, trudging through tasks, but mostly just sitting in her lounge in the warm darkness, waiting.

The referral came via her GP, a diligent doctor who carried out an impromptu home visit and was shocked at her decline. Although she'd been prescribed antidepressants, she remained low, nihilistic, crushingly depressed. Doing his job, the GP wondered if a specialist mental health team could offer anything he couldn't, and so referred to us.

When I told my manager that I'd known Jack as a trainee, she offered to allocate Mary's care coordination to another colleague. Situations like this happen – sometimes you discover patients live near you, you recognise them from your gym, or they dated someone you're mates with. There are no hard and fast rules, but generally, the less a patient knows about me specifically, the better.

I considered taking up this offer. In the end, I chose not to. I'd been working as a community mental health nurse for a while by this point and had supported some complex patients. I didn't get into this job for an easy ride. I wanted to help. But that wasn't all. A part of me was drawn to Mary. She was a link to Jack, the young man whose suicide I'd never fully reconciled.

So I rolled up my sleeves and dived in, visiting her weekly, applying the biopsychosocial model I'm now au fait with: the bio bit concerns any physical health supports that could be made, including medications being introduced, or signposting to general medicine; the psycho bit focuses on possible psychological therapy that could be trialled; and the social bit relates to any socio-environmental changes to improve the patient's quality of life.

For Mary, this meant arranging for a psychiatrist to carry out a home visit and tweak her antidepressants; he discussed diet, sleep and exercise too, and had the GP prescribe thiamine and ferrous sulfate as well as meal supplements; it meant facilitating a home visit from a clinical psychologist who posited the idea of bereavement therapy as something to consider to address unresolved grief; it meant initiating welfare checks to bump up Mary's entitlement of incapacity support, sourcing a cleaner who could help manage the large house, finding a charity for parents who've lost children.

All these things Mary accepted, but none had the impact I hoped for. She remains frozen in grief. So it is that we've ended up as we are now, sitting together, looking at the portrait of Jack above the mantle.

'I can't believe it,' she says. 'Five years. It's still not real.'

'I understand.'

She shakes her head again, smiling mournfully, and for the first time that day, her eyes find mine. 'No, you don't. Wait till you have one of your own. Then you might.'

Mary's right, of course – I don't understand loss of the kind she's experienced. Sure, I'd read books on suicide and risk assessing; I'd studied Durkheim, Camus, Plath; I know the shocking stats and demographics attached to these kinds of deaths, how suicide remains the biggest killer of young men, how certain professions like farmers and health workers have higher levels, and a family history of completed suicides will heighten risks. I know early warning signs for suicidality too – have a gut instinct for what to look out for; have even pre-empted an attempt that may've saved a patient's life.

But this is all surface, really, the anecdotal stuff to share with colleagues. Never has the terrible pain that comes from losing a child touched my life.

'I want a baby,' Clare says.

I look up. A moment ago, we were drinking foamy cappuccinos in our narrow galley kitchen, a morning routine before heading to our respective jobs.

'I've been thinking about it a lot. I'm sure.'

My eyes stay with hers, and then I look away and don't say anything.

She continues, 'I remember we talked about it a while back–'

'We did,' I say.

'But, well, I thought we could talk about it again.'

'Right,' I say, 'maybe later,' and I kiss her quickly, missing her lips, then race for the door.

Clare's right: we had talked about this, and I'd assumed the topic was dealt with. A couple of years prior, on holiday in Kraków, and after visiting the Auschwitz Concentration Camp site, I'd told Clare that I didn't want kids. I'd known for a while that parenthood wasn't something I was drawn to, and the haunting glimpse into the evil men are capable of, coupled with the knowledge that our relationship was becoming long term, compelled me to tell her.

'I figured you should know,' I said. 'Before we take things any further.'

Her face darkened, and she nodded.

And that should've been it.

By then, friends were beginning to breed. I saw the

sacrifices, the compromises, the repetition and bickering it brought to their relationships. Buggies and breast pumps, afternoon napping times and countless trips to swing parks filled me with dread. I liked being spontaneous, going to weird art shows, open-mic gigs, festivals; I wanted to travel, meet people and write. Not change nappies and go to soft-play and clip'N-climb.

There was more, though, behind my resistance; I see that now. The job had affected me. I'd met patients whose whole families perished in the Mogadishu bombings; I'd seen the ways kids can go off the rails – drugs, self-harm, mental illness; the world was unsafe, full of risks and hazards, predators and cruelty; I'd sat with parents like Mary who'd lost their kids to senseless deaths. Who'd bring a child into a world like this?

It forged a commitment to not have any of my own. Not because I don't like kids – actually, I enjoy their innocence, lack of sarcasm, their keen eyes and contagious laughs. But what if something went wrong? Like with Jack. How the hell would I live?

That night, over a lacklustre meal, Clare and I begin thrashing it out.

'Why complicate things? Isn't our life good?'

'It *is* good,' she says, 'and this could make it better.' She looks away. 'We've always been honest with each other.'

'Yes.'

'If we don't do this now, I don't know if we ever will.'

'Why?'

She lists off factors – how she's in her mid-thirties now, and the women in her family became perimenopausal early;

how she is in a place in her career where she's ready; and mostly, how her feelings about a baby have grown stronger.

'I want to be a mum,' she says.

I don't reply.

'You'd be a good dad.'

'How do you know?'

Over the next few days, we tussle, back-and-forth exchanges on the cusp of conflict that go nowhere; when not doing this, there are creeping silences, tiptoeing around the flat, our backs to each other in bed, the inches between us canyons.

I speak to friends, watch parents with newborns, try grafting my own life onto theirs. It doesn't look beyond the realms of possibility. But to own one of these things – a baby – and to call it mine? Terrifying.

By the same token, though, I can't fathom my life without Clare. I sense she will stay with me if we remain childless. But I also know that if she doesn't have this opportunity, a part of her will be sad, a sadness I have a part in.

So, I mull. I write my thoughts down. I study dads, trying to see with fresh eyes these hapless, harried, yet peculiarly happy men. I chat to a few. I listen. All say it's tiring, repetitive, how little free time they have. Yet none regret it.

Gradually, I find myself seeing it.

Me. With a baby.

Dad.

'OK,' I say to Clare a few nights later while we read in bed. She looks over.

'Let's do it.'

*

It proves easy to conceive.

We go through all the clichés – the positive pregnancy test photo on Facebook, announcements to grandparents-to-be, possible names, hospitals to give birth in. Each time we visit the mother and baby unit, I see the pomegranate object on the ultra-sound screen taking form, shape, a dot at its core pulsing.

My life takes on a strange duality: work and baby, work and baby. While I sit with my patients, asking when they'd last made plans to kill themselves, I think of this foetus, unspoiled, oblivious to life's hardships.

As Clare's belly grows, my workload grows too. The community mental health team I'm with has always been understaffed, but post-Brexit the shortfall is crippling. There are gaping holes in service delivery, vulnerable patients going weeks, months, without being seen. Two consultant psychiatrists are parachuted in as locums and both walk out within weeks, stating the service isn't fit for purpose; sickness levels spike, colleagues moan and berate and cry in toilets.

Meanwhile, Mary carries on staring at the picture of Jack, locked inside her quiet world. Of all my patients, she piques my fears about fatherhood the most.

When I visit her, I ask the usual questions, make chit-chat and avoid her half-masted eyes, saying nothing about my pending parenthood. And when I head home, and stare at Clare's tummy, I try to put Mary far from my thoughts. Focus on Erin – for it's a girl we'll be having.

We're on holiday in Morocco, trekking through the rugged terrain of the Atlas Mountains, when things go wrong.

Clare has some spotting. Bleeding isn't uncommon during pregnancy, and I do my best to reassure her that it'll be OK. But she already knows there's a problem. As do I.

The bleeds escalate, and on our return home, we head to the central London hospital where we planned for Clare to give birth. The obstetrician slicks her belly with gel and performs an ultrasound. And then it all comes crashing down. No heartbeat. Sometimes it happens, he says.

Suddenly, our world jolts to a halt. I look at Clare and she looks at me and neither of us knows what to say.

A strange kind of autopilot takes over. I book the taxi home, maintain the flat, bring Clare cups of tea, do the next thing I have to, then the next. We don't really talk. It's too raw. But in my heart, it's confirmation: having children carries risks.

Cruelly, Clare's second-trimester body still thinks she's pregnant, and it's doing what it's meant to do to see it through to completion. As such, the medics inform us that an abortion is needed to remove our daughter.

The following day, we sit together in the waiting lounge of the unit that deals with terminations. Alongside us are other pregnant women, some flicking through magazines, chewing gum, others furrowed and crying, all carrying foetuses they don't want, or can't keep.

After the process, a swift expunging I thankfully don't witness, Clare emerges from theatre pale and drawn, her belly already shrunk. I hold her hand and thank the staff.

We get another cab home.

A few months later, there's another miscarriage, preceded by the same red spotting, the wait for confirmation, and then the sense of powerlessness at hearing it.

Clare is devastated. Looking back, I see that I don't handle it too well. For a baby – a thing I didn't even want – has become the central focus of our life as a couple. It's as emotionally gruelling as my work. Clare has stockpiled books on fertility, gestation, enhancing the likelihood of seeing pregnancies through to completion. Blending and juicing, reducing caffeine, increasing vitamins, become military processes. Nothing feels fun anymore.

One day, I cautiously suggest that we might hit pause on 'project baby', take stock, remove a foot from the gas just for a bit.

'You're serious?' Clare says.

I turn away, aware of my mistake.

Clare's worked out her cycle like a da Vinci map, pinpointing exact times to do this, not do that, everything down to the finest minutiae.

I try to administer some mental health nursing skills on myself, exercising, getting enough sleep, practising mindfulness. Strangely, work becomes a refuge, a way to stay out of my own head and be in someone else's, albeit someone struggling with their own issues.

But in truth, I know I'm not handling things well. And it's about to get worse.

'She *may* make a full recovery,' the doe-eyed A&E registrar says to me, scanning through Mary's charts on the screen. 'But it's too soon to say. And her arm . . . well, it's not in a good way.'

I nod, uselessly.

'You're her care coordinator?'

'Yes,' I say.

'When did you last visit her?'

'A few weeks back.' It was more like four.

'Did you get a sense she might do something like this?'

'No,' I say, then hesitate, wracking my brain. Had I sensed Mary might try but ignored it? Was I too caught up in my own stuff to see the signs? 'Can I see her?'

'Sure,' the registrar says. 'Follow me.'

While we walk to the ward where she's been admitted, I'm given a summary. At some time in the last forty-eight hours, Mary took a staggered overdose of prescription pills. As they took effect, she must've slipped off her chair by the mantle where Jack's picture sits and come to rest on the carpet. Here, she rolled against the radiator that slowly baked her right arm.

By chance, a savvy carer I'd arranged to visit to help Mary with cleaning and shopping arrived early. The shrewd young Ghanaian woman persevered trying to get her client's attention, peering through the window, noticing what appeared to be a body. She called 999 and the police forced entry, saving Mary's life.

But when I see her, she looks dead. Supine on a hospital bed, wires feeding into and from her, her vitals displayed like a scene from *Casualty*. Her right arm is ensconced in bandages, horribly crooked; her lips are flaked and her pallor is chalk white.

'Mary,' I say.

Nothing.

I call her ex-husband Roger, Jack's dad, alerting him to what's happened. He's remarried, and his last contact with

Mary was a perfunctory exchange about the house that remains partially in his name. He thanks me for telling him, and then goes, not asking for the name of the hospital where she is. I try to contact other family members to no avail. Mary's parents are both dead and there's no siblings, friends, neighbours. Just me.

To try to make myself feel useful, I go about securing her home, ensuring the door that was rammed in gets boarded up, her valuables kept safe. The picture of Jack bales from above the mantle, his eyes following me like the Mona Lisa's.

That evening, I walk for hours, brooding, looking around the high street, passing fried chicken shops and second-hand electrical stores, hoping the distraction might alleviate this knot in me. I tell myself this wasn't my fault. Sure, the frequency of my visits to see Mary had decreased. But I hadn't committed a dereliction in my duty of care. In mental health, things like this happen. Deal with it, Sweeney.

But in my heart I know there was more I could've done. If I'd been more attentive, visited a week ago, read the non-verbal cues, this could've been avoided. The certainty leaves me on edge. Right now, this world seems a mean place.

And I'm thinking about bringing a child into it?

Mary spends several weeks on a general ward. Doctors attend to her arm and monitor her liver function after the pounding her overdose gave it. Once stable, she's conveyed to a mental health unit, situated at the same site but on a different ward from where Jack spent time all those years back. She spends three months here, detained on a section of the Mental Health Act due to the risk of further attempts on her life.

I visit several times. It's a busy ward, always with a few howling patients pacing up and down the corridors. Her room has the familiar washed-out effect, beige, bland walls, grubby handprints, the prerequisite suicide-resistant fixtures and fittings. The lead psychiatrist has upped her meds and Mary has had a couple of sessions with a psychologist – progress. We agree that she will always present a risk to herself, but we can't keep her locked up forever.

Approaching her discharge date, I visit again. Mary has positioned her chair by the window. She wears a dressing gown and slippers and sits there, cradling her lame arm, her eyes hooded, staring at her phone and the photo of Jack she has saved.

'What do you think he would've made of all this?' she whispers, her voice husky.

I take my time. 'I think he'd have been sad. To know that you've had a rough time.'

'What must you think of me, causing all this bother?'

'It's no bother,' I say. 'I'm just glad you're still here.' We are quiet a moment. Somewhere, a patient groans, and an alarm beeps.

'What about you?' Mary says. 'Are you OK?'

I look up, realise her eyes are on me. 'Why do you ask?' I say.

'I may be batty, but I was a mum once. I know when something's wrong.'

'I'm fine,' I say. It's my first real lie to a patient.

*

Clare is pregnant again. We went through the standard fare of shock, hugging, crying and silence. By now, we're versed in this pantomime and agree to keep the news between ourselves and see what happens. If things go wrong, at least it'll just be us dealing with it.

But things don't go wrong. Instead, Clare reaches trimester two, then approaches the third and final stage. It's strange, watching her grow again, like revisiting a book I've already read but with an unfinished third act. When the bump really starts showing, she begins telling a few friends, her parents, and things get real.

A baby.

We go to antenatal classes and NCT groups, vaccine talks, the John Lewis buggy department, where forlorn fathers-to-be traipse behind pregnant partners. I try to appear eager, the way expectant parents should, but inside there's a numbness masking my fear.

Scans show that we're having a boy this time. Tentatively, we list possible names. Jack crosses my mind and is a contender. In the end we opt for Spencer, my favourite literary private investigator, albeit spelled the more conventional way.

Keep calm and carry on. That's what I tell myself. But as Clare approaches full term, something in me feels it is broiling, going astray. A few days later, on a baking morning in June, I find myself breaking all the professional boundary rules, sharing with the most inappropriate person: Mary.

She's been discharged from hospital now for several weeks and we're back at her house. Adaptations have been fitted – shower rails, kitchen guards – to accommodate for her disabled arm, which the medics managed to save but will never have normal function.

Despite this, the stay in hospital seems to have been beneficial – colour has returned to her cheeks and she's put on some much-needed weight. This in turn has made her more chatty, affable, able to engage. She still carries that pall of sadness and her eyes reflexively flit to the picture of Jack, but there is a vigour to her that was absent before.

I can't remember what triggers the chat. From memory she commented again about me not seeming quite right. This time, I just didn't have it in me to lie. So I tell her.

'I'm going to be a dad.'

There's no way to retract it. This is a patient, a woman whose only son took his life, and who came close to ending her own. I'm disclosing the most personal thing in my life, and quite possibly the thing that could trigger her most. Am I mad?

'Sorry,' I say.

'Why are you?' she says.

'I shouldn't have said that.'

Mary's face takes on an inwardness, like she's working out a sum. She looks at Jack as if he might know the answer. Then she looks back at me, leans in and says, 'Good.'

'Good?'

She nods. 'Now you'll understand.' Her grey eyes are suddenly lit up. 'Aren't you happy?'

Happy? Stressed. Scared. Unhinged. But happy wasn't a word I'd considered.

'I don't know,' I say.

She nods again. 'My husband was the same. Just wait till you hold that little baby, though. Then you will be.'

Slants of grey light fillet through the gaps in the blind, sparkling off her glistening cheeks.

She's crying.

So am I.

Sweet and Tender Hooligan

A FEW MINUTES before 8 a.m. on a Friday morning in mid-June, Neville, forty-four, pulls his hood up over his dreads, adjusts his wraparound shades, takes a deep breath and boards the Victoria Line train among heaving rush-hour commuters, all headed northbound. There are no seats, hardly anywhere to stand, bodies crammed against bodies, a pressure cooker. Each nerve fibre in Neville screams to flee.

But he can't – this is too important. He grabs the handrail with one hand, waits for the doors to close, the carriage to grumble to life. Then he exhales. A woman listening to headphones stares up. Glares more like. Does she know him? Suspect what he's doing? Instinctively, Neville reaches into his pocket . . .

She looks away. False alarm.

Neville steadies. He must stay calm. Glares he can handle. He's had to put up with a lot worse since his life began to unravel and they started locking him up in prison cells, so-called hospitals, and that bogus psychiatrist prescribed those mind-control pills.

Not anymore. Now, Neville's awake. He understands.

A bead runs down his forehead. It's hot as hell and he can smell his sweat. Hardly surprising. After he walked out of his flat last Tuesday, going dark, he's been in these same clothes, wandering back alleys, public parks, sleeping on benches and buses, staying alert. Somewhere along the way he lost his shoe – he can't recall how, maybe they stole it – but he knows for sure his phone and wallet were nicked while he was dozing. Seized would be the more accurate term. By agents. He won't let that happen again.

Those first few nights he was running scared, sure he would come a cropper. They'd find him. Stage his death. Make it look like natural causes. You read about these stories: body of unknown man found; no foul play suspected. Well, they won't get Neville that easily. After today, the world will know the truth and–

Metal screeches and the train grinds to a halt. Passengers lurch. Someone elbows Neville. An agent? He tenses, reaches into his pocket again, touches the round hilt of the penknife. He's ready to defend, attack, even turn the weapon on himself to evade torture.

Silence. Neville studies faces, his heart in his throat.

Then the driver's voice through a speaker: 'Morning, ladies and gents, apologies for the delay . . .' Something about signal failure. Nothing to worry about.

Neville grins. False alarm.

This driver though, he's speaking with an accent. Russian? Relief becomes renewed panic. The air is sucked

SWEET AND TENDER HOOLIGAN

from Neville's chest. The train chugs back to life. Don't be daft, he reasons. It's not an agent. Just a train driver. Get a grip. Neville chuckles, realising his mind is playing tricks. The headphones woman glares again. Neville covers his mouth to stifle the noise.

Who'd have guessed he'd end up like this? All he ever wanted was a normal life. For a few years, after the horror in the army, he had it: his own plumbing business, a missus, a flat, a baby girl. Where did it go so wrong? Why did his life fall so precipitously away?

Soon, they will arrive at Victoria. A change to the Circle Line, then it's a short walk to the Russian Embassy . . .

At Oxford Circus, people get off, more get on. Tourists. Businessmen. Parents and kids. Neville scans them. No one suspicious. But the woman with headphones still hasn't moved. He can hear the *tsh-tsh-tsh* from her music. He's sure he recognises the song. Rihanna. One of his daughter's favourites. Is this a way to taunt him?

At the thought of Cristina, something crushes in his heart. He shakes his head, rids the memory away. Stay strong. He's doing this for her. He looks for a divergence, reading the adverts by the air vents. Cures for male-pattern baldness. Apps for life insurance quotes. PPE reimbursement calculators. All strange, nonsensical. Ridiculous slogans. Yet *not* random. The more Neville takes them in, the more he sees sequences there. Subliminal messages. Codes. Surely these can't have been tampered with too?

A spider of fear begins crawling up his spine. This time, he can't shake it off. What if the Russians figured out a way to infiltrate Transport for London? They're on this train now.

Is there nowhere safe? The realisation makes his knees turn to jelly. How in God's name can he go against an enemy this sophisticated?

That's when he makes his mistake. He starts chuckling again. At how ludicrous, how impossible his mission is. He's one man against the system. It turns into full-blown laughter. He can't stop.

Neville hears his bellows filling the carriage and knows it's too late. He puts his hand over his mouth. That just makes it worse. Laughter spills out like molten lava. Soon, they'll lock him up. They'll hurt him. Make him talk.

'No,' he says between bursts, and finds the penknife. 'No, not that.'

Tears stream from his eyes. He rubs his cheek. His shades topple onto the floor. He can't stop laughing.

It's futile. Everything's lost. All Neville can do is laugh and laugh. He tried. But he failed, like he failed everything, and he doesn't know what's happening anymore. Everyone's looking, they're all in on it, of course they are, and he feels like his head really is about to go 'Pop!' like a cartoon character and—

Someone touching him. A hand on his arm.

Neville starts pulling the penknife out.

He sees it's the woman with the headphones. Only she's removed them now. She's looking at him. Kind eyes. Concerned. But can he trust her? Can he?

'Are you OK?' she says.

'I . . .' Neville says, and falters.

He has no idea what to say.

*

SWEET AND TENDER HOOLIGAN

Some of this I learn from the British Transport Police who attended the platform after reports of a disturbed male with a knife came through; some of it I read in Neville's clinical notes that describe his recent release from prison for shoplifting, subsequent disengagement with his psychiatrist and his point-blank refusal to accept medication for his illness; some of it I was told by his ex-partner Olive, mum of his daughter Cristina, who'd had to draw a line with Neville recently because his beliefs and broken promises became too much; but most I gleaned from Neville himself when I spoke with him a few hours later.

We're in the basement of a central London hospital, a segregated area known as a 'health-based place of safety'. There's little that feels safe here: it's more akin to a world war bunker, hidden deep underground, with a foreboding sense of incarceration. Three secure rooms – cells might be a more accurate term – are each occupied by disgruntled-looking patients visible through thick cracked screens.

One rotund Asian woman has refused to tell the staff who she is, and sits with her face to the wall, mute. A thin black man doesn't appear to know who he is, and lies on his cot, crying and bleating. Neville occupies the room at the end. He's slumped by the wall, thick knees hugged close to his wide chest. He stares through his dreads.

All three of these people have different backstories. What unifies them is they have each been scooped up by the police and brought here to be assessed under the Mental Health Act.

Some effort has been made to brighten the space with wall-mounted beach prints, and an air diffuser pumps out wafts of chemically floral scent. But it all feels like a nicotine chewing gum, minty and fresh on the surface but masking a bitter aftertaste.

Outside the rooms, two stocky security guards sit on fold-up chairs, both immersed in their smartphones. Opposite the guards, cramped in a broom-cupboard office, two tired nurses are on stools behind desktops. They are both attacking keyboards, typing up their observation notes about these three patients, what they've eaten, drank, said, not said.

With Neville, the write-ups are meagre. Since he arrived here a few minutes after ten in the morning, he's not said or done a thing.

Neville's an ex-serviceman, and his experiences of trauma and institutional racism growing up, and then in the army, are contributory factors that led to his mental ill health. Combine these with an absent father, significant amounts of cannabis use as a teenager, and a family history of paranoid schizophrenia on his mother's side, and the odds were stacked against him. When well, he's affable, funny, easy-going; when poorly, he's a risk to others and himself, and can't be ignored.

I've met Neville once before, about a year back, in a situation much like this. Police had been called after he was seen acting bizarrely in a shopping centre, brandishing a knife, which led to them tasering him and piling in rugby-tackle style. I'd only just come back from two weeks of paternity leave. My head had been full of baby-speak, the smell of nappy cream, the jingle of 'Rock-a-Bye Baby' on repeat. I returned to work happy, albeit tired, and with hope. Seeing Neville's raw bruises, grazed knuckles and his psychosis in full flight were enough to catapult me back to the grim reality of acute mental health.

There's a predictable pattern to Neville's lapses – first, he stops his involvement with his community mental health team, eschewing his antipsychotic meds because of side-effects, deciding he doesn't need any of that claptrap, he can go it alone; before long, he becomes persecuted, sure that nefarious forces are conspiring to thwart him; shortly after this, Neville starts plotting, conjuring ways to usurp said forces by whatever means. This includes the use of weapons, committing criminal acts, assaults, planned attacks. He's walloped strangers staring at him, sent vexatious threats to public figures, chased children, and has had several stints in prison as well as a year in Broadmoor. In this sense, he falls into a minority of patients who generate a huge amount of panic and notoriety – mentally disordered offenders.

Today, the British Transport Police have placed Neville on a section 136 of the Mental Health Act. This allows a constable to bring a person they believe is suffering a mental health crisis to a secure setting for up to twenty-four hours, during which time they are to be assessed.

By now, police procedural terms like this are familiar to me: as well as being a registered nurse, I've become an approved mental health professional, trained in the use of the Mental Health Act. The Act is the medical-legal interface that provides a framework for certain patients to be detained to hospital to be assessed and treated, whether they consent or not. It's a meaty piece of statute, overlapping with the Equality Act, the Mental Capacity Act, and, as its backbone, the Human Rights Act.

Although the Mental Health Act has gone through several revisions over the decades since its first passing, it has always been a contentious piece of legislation, and perhaps should be. For it makes deprivation of liberty and forceable treatment legal. In Neville's case, this will likely involve four nurses pinning him down and a fifth jabbing his bum with a syringe full of antipsychotics. Imagine it. In a different context, this would be considered assault.

I've jousted with people who see the Act as draconian, oppressive, cruel, a way to legitimise the removal of society's undesirables because of the majority's intolerances. They argue that it tars the mentally ill with the same brush as criminals, then labels them with diagnoses that lead them to be shovelled with potent drugs to keep them controlled. I do have sympathy with this argument: the Nursing and Midwifery Council Code of Practice provides a list of standards all nurses, midwives and nurse associates must adhere to. Words like kindness, respect, empowerment, individual choice and diversity fill its pages. Not detention, compulsion and restraint.

My answer to critics of the Act is, what's the alternative? Sadly, there's a minority of patients for whom detention is the only port of call. Some might hurt themselves through self-neglect or self-harm; some are a risk to others due to paranoia and delusions. Neville ticks all these boxes. Would you really want him wandering the streets near you in his present state?

'Ahem,' I say.

One of the security guards looks up from Candy Crush on his phone. The other doesn't register.

I point at Neville.

SWEET AND TENDER HOOLIGAN

The one paying attention sighs to a stand, withdraws a bundle of keys, checks his pepper spray cannister strapped to his belt. Then he unlocks Neville's room.

As the door opens, the smell wafts out – musty sweat from Neville's filthy clothes, his barefoot, unclean body and a lingering hangover from previous occupiers. Some new clothes have been left on the wall-affixed cot – the standard lime-green tunic and pants – but Neville's refused them, no doubt suspecting they've been tampered with. From the floor, he stares up.

'Hello, Neville,' I say, staying in the doorway, ready to retreat should he move suddenly. 'We're here from the mental health team. Can we speak to you?'

The stare remains.

'I've met you before,' I say, 'and my two colleagues have too.' I gesture at two doctors to my rear.

Chloe, a sleep-deprived, middle-grade psychiatrist, on call for every mental health patient within this hospital, flashes her ID, says 'Hi' coolly, officiously; Dr Barr, Neville's community psychiatrist, who has an important lecture to deliver later that morning to a hall of postgrads, gives a wide, false smile.

'You're working for them,' Neville says.

'For who?' I say.

'Go away.'

'Why've you not been taking your medication, Neville?' Dr Barr says, a schoolmaster tone to his voice. 'We've been in this situation before.'

''Cause I don't need it. It's poison. There's nothin' wrong with me.'

'Let's have a chat about that,' I say.

Neville says nothing.

'Well,' Dr Barr says, 'what's the issue with the medication this time?'

'The *issue*?' Nev says, mimicking the psychiatrist's enunciation, 'is that you lot think I'm crazy.'

'We don't use words like crazy,' Dr Barr says, checking the time on his Rolex. 'Mentally ill, perhaps.'

'Who're you to say I'm mentally ill?'

'Well, I'm a consultant psychiatrist.'

'No you're not.'

'It's me who prescribes the medication which you've persistently refused to take. If you came to appointments, I'd explain why you need them and consider alternatives, but I've not seen you in months. And now you're here.'

Neville shakes his head. 'You're all in on it.'

Dr Barr leans over to me. Conspiratorially, he says: 'He's paranoid, like last time. I don't think there's much point carrying on—'

'I want to get out of here!' Neville screams, spittle flying from his mouth. 'You can't keep me locked up like a dog!'

The two guards step around us, hands on their pepper spray cans like gunslingers.

'Easy,' I say.

Neville breathes heavily, staring up. He stares and stares and then lowers his chin to his hands. Tears plop onto his dirty bare feet.

'Thank you, Neville,' Dr Barr says. Turning to me, he again says, 'Not much point carrying on.' He glances at his

Rolex a second time, less conspicuously. 'He's too far gone. We need to section him.'

To section somebody, we must all agree it's in the patient's best interests. Here, I suspect Dr Barr is right: Neville is clearly unwell. But I'm not done yet. I step forward. The security guards shuffle together, but I manoeuvre around them. Seeing me, Neville's body tightens like a fist.

Crouching, I say, 'I spoke to your ex-wife. She's worried. So's your daughter. Cristina.'

He says nothing.

'What happened? How'd you get yourself like this?'

'I can't talk about it. Don't know who you are.'

'Is it possible you're not too well?'

Another, longer pause.

It spills out of him then, like steam through a vent. How he stopped the meds during his last stint in prison because they made him drowsy and meant he couldn't take his daughter to school when he came out; how he decided to drop out of the mental health team, the probation worker, ignore their poxy phone calls and the appointments with Dr Barr; he was going to have a normal life, and started getting his energy back, feeling more like old Neville . . . until the spies started appearing, the symbols, the messages, all part of an elaborate plot.

For twenty long minutes he continues like this, the tears streaming as he speaks. Much of what he says is pressurised, persecutory, nonsensical, chopped-up paragraphs lifted from a breakneck spy novel all blurted out; but beneath the crackle and static of paranoia, I hear the pathos of a human in pain. It's this I try to focus on.

'I want to leave this place now,' he says at the end. 'I need to go.'

I look at both doctors. Chloe watches, wet-eyed. Dr Barr is immersed in his phone.

'Neville,' I ask, 'where would you go?'

He wipes his runny nose. 'I'd go back out on the street. I can't go home. Not safe.'

'Would you be willing to see Dr Barr and people from his team? Maybe go back onto your meds?'

'Haven't you been listening to a word I said?'

'I have. But I think a lot of what you're experiencing is caused by a mental illness. It's making you have thoughts and feelings that aren't real. What do you reckon?'

He shakes his head wearily, like he was expecting this. 'It's real,' he says. 'They've got to you.'

Dr Barr clears his throat. I ignore him.

'OK,' I say. 'I'm going to have a chat with the doctors.' I push to a stand. 'Then I'll come back and talk to you.'

Neville stares up. He hesitates and then holds out his hand for me to shake. A large hand. Capable of strength. The nails long, darkened with dirt and grit. Dr Barr wouldn't shake that hand, and I don't much want to; but to refuse this small act of human connection seems wrong.

'Let's get you a cuppa and some food into you,' I say, as his warm dry fingers enclave my palm.

The support and management of the Nevilles of this country is a challenge for all of us, professionals and the public alike. The simplistic label – defining a patient as either mad, bad or sad – fails to encapsulate the complexities in this client group, where overlaps between the mental health and criminal justice systems seem fuzzy, and maintaining patient and public safety even fuzzier.

The riskiest patients are sometimes detained to medium-secure or even special hospitals – Ashworth, Rampton or Broadmoor being the three infamous ones in the UK. Here, aggression and antisociality are generally viewed as symptoms of mental disorder. There are no fixed length stays in these places; discharge is a complex process, determined by doctors and the Home Office, requiring close social supervision and monitoring.

Others, though, will languish in prisons, serving sentences, punished for actions deemed to be criminal behaviour; they're locked up in overcrowded, understaffed institutions teeming with aggression. Charlie Taylor, chief inspector of prisons in the UK, published recent data indicating the soaring rates of self-harm, drug use and suicide attempts in the prison estate – people go in with a BA in pot smoking and moderate anxiety and come out with a PhD in crack use and suicidal ideation.

Many, like Neville, flit between these two sectors, spending time subject to the criminal and mental health frameworks. Ronnie Kray and Ian Brady, two of the twentieth century's most notorious offenders, both had diagnosed mental illnesses, both committed serious crimes and both spent time in prison and hospital. The perception from the public can be that the professionals don't know what they're doing. Perhaps they're right.

High-profile tragedies where mentally disordered offenders commit heinous crimes garner interest. But instead of creating solutions, these rare events are like flies under a magnifying glass. Quickly, members of the public fear that *all* mentally unwell people are dangerous, and we're putting society at risk by letting any of them roam the streets.

The Christopher Clunis Enquiry from the mid-1990s was my first encounter of this kind of furore. Following the murder of musician Andrew Zito, a damning report listed the missed opportunities among public services that allowed Clunis, a paranoid schizophrenic with a clear history of offending, to be left unsupported and unsupervised, until tragedy struck.

Clunis murdered Zito, a stranger, at Finsbury Park tube station, close to where I was brought up, and was detained for the remainder of his life, dying in hospital. I remember his image in the tabloids, cropped to emphasise his large, menacing eyes, unrepentant expression, his fearsome size. The fact that he was an African-Caribbean man who'd killed a Caucasian can't be ignored either, for racism was, and is, inherent in psychiatry, and the thought of a black schizophrenic rampaging around seems to tap into a certain kind of public outrage.

Three decades on, and it's sometimes hard to see evidence of improvements. Parallels between Clunis and Valdo Calocane, the 2023 Nottingham stabber, are glaring, as are the missed opportunities to have intervened with him sooner. Calocane, also a black schizophrenic with a track record of violence when unwell, disengaged from his mental health team, wasn't assertively pursued, and went on to stab to death three strangers and injure more while in a psychotic state. The press images of his mugshot are eerily akin to Clunis's, showing the flat eyes of a monster. I suspect if Neville had perpetrated a violent act, the powers that be would have unearthed a comparable shot of him.

In the broom-cupboard office, the two nurses shuffle out to make space, and the two doctors and I enter and decide what happens next.

A post-interview discussion is a vital part of a Mental Health Act assessment. All three of us need to agree that less restrictive options have been exhausted, and to admit Neville would be in his best interests, or the interests of the public. These meetings can trigger lively debates and, occasionally, clashes. This is a good thing, for when the stakes are high and we're proposing detaining someone, matters should be thrashed out fully.

Dr Barr has made up his mind. 'He's unwell. Simple as that. Mad as a box of frogs. No insight. Doesn't think he's got a mental illness. He needs to go into hospital pronto.' He removes a pen from his suit pocket, looks at me. 'Have you got any section papers?'

'Hold on,' I say, his enthusiasm to get Neville carted off grating. I turn to Chloe. 'What do you think?'

She shrugs, looks at Dr Barr, at me, and nods. 'I can't see any other options. Neville's in crisis, and he doesn't recognise it. If we let him go, he'll be back on the street, refusing treatment, putting himself and the public at risk.'

She's right. Neville's too caught up in his delusions to be able to accept help. If there'd been interventions sooner, an assertive effort to get him back on his meds, perhaps this could've been avoided; but it's too late, the intensity of his paranoia and his certainty that he doesn't have a mental illness blocking the chances to support him in a community setting.

It's a familiar story. Why does it happen? Where to start? There's the chronic lack of resources in mental health services, along with poor multiagency communication between the NHS, social care, criminal justice and voluntary sectors; there's the understaffing in mental health teams, leading to demotivation, apathy, corner cutting, complacency; and there's the fear that patients like Neville generate: loud, scary men known to shout and wave knives.

In Neville's case, another cause is the support – or lack of – he's been given. Dr Barr might take a libertarian view, stating that by letting him disengage and stop taking his antipsychotic meds, he was respecting his wishes. For me, this won't wash. If Dr Barr had rolled up his sleeves and gone out to see Neville to try to persuade him round, we might not be here.

Now options are limited. We have a very ill man, and we can't let him go.

'You agree then?' Dr Barr says to me, a little tetchily. 'He's coming in?'

I nod.

'There we have it. It's sad, but inevitable. Patients like him *do* get ill and go a little . . .' He taps his head demonstratively.

'Crazy?' I say.

Dr Barr smiles, but the smile fades when he sees my expression.

In silence, I dig out a Section Two recommendation for the doctors to complete. These benign, pink-coloured sheets allow Neville's freedom to be removed for up to twenty-eight days.

As Dr Barr begins writing, he says, 'Patients need to take responsibility for their mental health. He knows he's ill. That's that.' A final check of the Rolex. 'Goodness, I must fly.'

I count to ten. Without doubt, Dr Barr is an eminent psychiatrist; I'm sure I'd be rapt listening to him lecture, and he'd make delightful company at a dinner party. But he's paid to do a job – albeit a tough one – to care for some of society's most downtrodden. Here, I suspect his eyes have fallen off the ball.

Now, Neville is getting sectioned. He'll struggle in hospital. Research shows that as an African-Caribbean man, the likelihood of him being restrained and having meds forced into him are significantly higher than in others. Traumas he's suffered in the past will be exhumed, and his mistrust for mental health staff will calcify even more. Meanwhile, Dr Barr will be waxing with his postgrads.

I consider saying something to this effect, but resist – no doubt it will end in a confrontation, a 'How dare you!' standoff that would detract from the task at hand – to help Neville.

'There,' Dr Barr says, handing me the section paper to scrutinise. 'May I go?'

His handwriting is barely legible, the curves and swirls of the lettering as condescending as his smile. I notice he's misspelled Neville's name. As he's halfway out the door, I point this out and suggest he rewrite it, printing his words for ease of eligibility.

'I'm in a rush,' he winces.

'Sorry,' I say, and smile.

*

It would be easy – *too* easy – to blame Neville's decline solely on Dr Barr, but this psychiatrist's laissez-faire attitude isn't isolated and represents a sad reality. Embedded in the UK mental health workforce there are levels of incompetence and disregard that continue to shock and depress me. I've seen instances of assumption making, prejudice and laziness from health care assistants, nurses, psychologists and medics, more interested in publishing papers and booking holidays than doing some good.

In mental health, it's not hard to get away with bad practice. If I insist a patient swears at me, threatens me or refuses to engage, it's doubtful I'll be challenged. Meanwhile, if a patient says I've done the same to them, it's easy to quash these claims as ramblings. These are, after all, crazy people.

Some mental health staff have been in it too long or have just run out of steam. They should probably hang up their lanyards too, do something else. But on top of the shirkers, there are those whose drives are pure schadenfreude. Recent BBC investigations have shone a spotlight on extreme instances of inpatient neglect and abuses of power. These, I hope, are rare, yet somewhere in the country right now, they will be happening.

Why are these people working in the sector in the first place? For some, there's an attraction, a delight in exercising control, pulling strings. Then, when things go wrong, to blame it on the patient.

I've known nurses sleep in the office when they should be observing volatile, dangerous men; doctors discharging abused women and then approaching them on dating apps, having sexual frissons in exchange for their 'help'. I've seen shocking stigma and, occasionally, downright lying to cover up failures and incompetencies.

'How a society treats its most vulnerable is always a measure of its humanity,' stated Ambassador Matthew Rycroft to the UN in 2014. On the strength of the UK mental health system, it's sometimes hard not to despair.

After the doctors have left I stay with Neville, waiting until news of a bed arrives. He continues staring. His two neighbours do the same. The nurses return to the office, the security guards to their phones.

Finding a suitable bed for a patient is an arduous process. Since the late 1980s, the number of inpatient psychiatric beds has dropped by approximately a third, while levels of mental illness have spiked, with a massive 34 per cent rise in detentions under the Mental Health Act. Now hundreds of patients wait hours, days, sometimes weeks for a suitable bed to be sourced, and are then sent to hospitals miles from their homes and communities due to local shortages, meaning family and friends will struggle to visit them.

On this occasion, Neville lands lucky. The patient flow manager informs me there's a male bed on a PICU (psychiatric intensive care unit) in one of the big hospitals a few miles away. The ambulance will be arriving shortly.

I go back into the room and tell Neville the news. He takes it badly, standing, stepping between me and the light slanting in from the barred window, his face dropping into shadow. Suddenly, he's galloping for me.

Fast, I exit the room, my heart pounding. The security

guards lock the door. Neville begins banging, screaming about the Russians, agents, conspiracies which I'm now involved with. He punches the glass repeatedly, crying and raging.

Eventually, he runs out of steam and placates. The wheels have fallen off. He slumps in a heap. 'I thought you were on my side,' he says, looking up, his breath clouding the glass.

'I am,' I say, enunciating loudly, so he can hear.

He shakes his head. 'I don't want to go back to hospital.'

'Why don't you?'

He takes a breath. I'm expecting a second wave of banging. 'Because I'm afraid.'

Sending Neville to hospital might not help in the long term. Sure, they'll put him back onto his antipsychotic meds, clean him up, make sure he and the public are safe. But then what? Upon discharge, there's a good chance he will disengage from mental health services, come off the meds, and the Russians will begin stalking him again. He'll decline further, lose any hope of building a relationship with his daughter, and maybe do something awful. It's too soon to know. Right now, all I can say is I've done my best for him with the resources I have.

Four burly ambulance drivers who could each be extras from *Prison Break* rock up.

Surrounding Neville, wary of sudden moves, they walk him from his cell, upstairs towards an unmarked ambulance with a celled rear cabin. At one point, I'm sure he's about to try and make a run for it. Instead, he scrunches his large frame into the small seat to the rear of the vehicle and stares at me until the doors are shut.

I watch the ambulance immerse into rush hour traffic. He's gone.

After typing my notes, firing out a report and contacting Neville's ex-wife, I head home. It's baking outside, a dry, savage kind of heat in a summer that kicked off with the Grenfell Tower fire.

Back home, our little flat, once neat and ordered, has become a swamp of buggies and sterilisers, carrycots and nappy bags. At times it feels overwhelmingly cluttered, but then I'm welcomed by the coos of Spencer, fast approaching one, and my anxiety is sated.

His arrival wasn't the seamless delivery we'd hoped for. Clare's waters broke in the small hours and, after zipping to hospital, our finely tuned birth plan fell astray. Midwives, obstetricians, health care assistants came and went, and Clare was trundled from cubicle to cubicle, stretcher to stretcher, then to the operating room, her legs akimbo, more midwives and medics coming and going, contradicting each other, the mantra of 'Push' the only constant.

Spencer came out purple and bruised, a searing curve scoring his face temple to chin where the forceps gripped him. I was allowed to cut the umbilical cord. It was tough and leathery and made me feel nauseous. Then I was handed a white towel from which stared a pair of marble eyes. My son. Nothing would ever be the same.

'How was your day?' Clare asks as I walk into the lounge. Spencer, in just a nappy, lays on her front, his brilliant eyes beaming.

'Fine,' I reply. Clare knows not to pry. I cannot possibly

describe the toil of what I've witnessed today without bringing us both down.

Instead, I bend over for Spencer, carefully lift him up, place my thumb in his wrinkly palm. His fingers grapple me. He gazes up. I think of Neville and his daughter and wonder if he did the same with her in those big, cracked hands.

'How are you?' I say.

Spencer licks his lips.

If this little boy grows up and says he'd like to be a mental health nurse like me, I'd be a proud dad.

But I'd be afraid too.

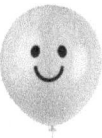

Girl Afraid

'Sorry,' Bobby says, looking at the floor, and then up at me. 'This is the last time.'

'That's what you said last time,' I say.

'But I mean it now.' She slurps from her Coke can and smiles ruefully.

It's mid-afternoon, and we're in the canteen area of the same north London hospital where I was born. Bobby, a few hours earlier, had walked into the A&E department; in full view of patients and staff, she sat on the floor, tied a ventilation tube fashioned into a noose around her neck and shouted that she planned to kill herself unless someone came and helped her.

Staff here, who know Bobby well due to the frequency of her visits, initially ignored the threat and carried on with their shift. Sometimes, Bobby grew bored and left of her own volition. On this occasion, she wasn't backing down. Bobby stayed put and tightened the noose.

Security got called, but by the time they arrived, Bobby

was golf ball-eyed, turning blue, and the ligature had to be severed with cutters. Reluctantly, nursing staff took her to one of the sole remaining cubicles, where she gasped and grinned like an alcoholic after a sneaky drink.

While a medic checked her vitals, confirmed that apart from a 360-indent circumnavigating her neck there was no permanent damage, a charge nurse called the on-site mental health liaison team, who in turn called me, Bobby's care coordinator, to come and deal with her.

'How are you feeling?' I ask.

'Better,' Bobby says, rubbing her neck where the indent is still visible.

'We agreed that you'd *not* do this. If you're feeling out of control, you're to practice your distraction techniques. If they don't work, call me. Remember?'

'I tried to call,' she says. 'You didn't pick up.'

'I was with another patient. I called you back as soon as I saw you'd rung.'

'Which patient were you with?'

'That's none of your business.'

'Are they as complex as me?'

'Same answer.'

'Hm.'

Bobby takes another slurp. I stare at her, dismally, trying to piece together how it came to this.

At twenty-six, it's a miracle she's still with us, for throughout her adolescence and adulthood she's been flirting with self-destruction, at times coming perilously close to taking things too far. There've been dozens of ligatures, climbing onto bridges, deep lacerations to arms and legs, overdoses, bleach, staple and nail swallowing, not to mention the insertions of foreign objects into orifices that even a seasoned mental health professional like me is shocked by.

Five-eight, plump and ruddy, she still dresses like a kid – Reeboks, Under Armour trackie, a Yankees' cap. Her body reads like a misery map, scudded with burns and scars, missing hair, chipped teeth, deep crows' feet around the eyes, the nose cratered and bent, her skin nicked and dinted as an old car bonnet. She talks like an extra from *Top Boy*, 'Cuz' this and 'Fam' that, acting the mean girl; but behind the front I've caught glimpses of a reservoir of sadness, unruly and unresolved too.

'Want to talk about what happened?' I say.

A Pinteresque pause; Bobby says, 'I was bored.'

'Bored?' Anger scratches at me. 'Why not read a book? Do the ironing?'

'Maybe.'

'Bobby,' I say, trying to look assertive, not exhausted, 'help me out here. You're going to end up dead at this rate. How can we keep this from happening so often?'

She puts her Coke on the floor, pulls out a pouch of tobacco and a Rizla, and begins rolling a cigarette. As her sleeve slides up, I catch sight of the scars, old and new, marring the skin haphazardly like the scribbling, scrawling artworks my son has started to produce.

'This is the last time,' she repeats.

'Really?'

'Really.'

Right now, Bobby seems steady. I want to believe what she's saying. But when you exist on the borderline between this and explosive, it takes little more than a dodgy look to tip you over.

'I'm going for a fag,' she says.

I nod.

'Coming?'

'No thanks.'

'Suit yourself.'

She stands, heads for the exit on the ground floor. Halfway down the escalator, she looks back. Her eyes find mine. I see it then, the wounded child in her, checking I'm still there, the way Spencer, my boy, does with me. How the hell did it get like this?

'Enjoy your smoke,' I say to no one, and chuck her Coke can in the bin.

Two hours later, as I'm getting home, I get another call from the hospital. Bobby has placed herself in front of fast-moving traffic on the A1. Police are bringing her back to A&E. She's asked the staff to call me.

According to NHS England, someone with a personality disorder will think, feel, behave and relate to others differently from the average person. Symptoms will depend on the type of personality disorder – PD for short – they are diagnosed with, its veracity, severity and how the PD manifests into their life.

Vague, isn't it?

What's clear is that these are some of the most maligned and misunderstood patients in mental health care. Staff can be left feeling useless, traumatised, angered, enraged. I certainly feel it working with Bobby.

At one time, a personality disorder was considered more a social issue than a clinical one. People demonstrating destructive, impulsive behaviours were signposted towards public services: drug and alcohol drop-ins, charities, peer support, the Samaritans, even the Church. The original Mental Health Act definitions made no mention of personality disorder, the closest being the term 'psychopathic disorder', meaning a 'persistent disorder or disability of the mind', reserved for those deemed to be high risk and incurable.

Gradually the definitions broadened. For what couldn't be refuted was the growing number of people presenting to services with emotional and behavioural difficulties, as well as the hugely detrimental impact said difficulties were having on their lives and on those around them. Eventually, this led to a new category of mental illness being classified – the personality disorders. And since then the numbers have bloomed.

During training we learned how personality disorders were divided into clusters: cluster A includes the odd/eccentric patients, paranoid, schizoid and schizotypal; cluster B, the emotionally dysregulated types, antisocial, borderline, histrionic, narcissistic; and cluster C covers the disorders anchored by fear – dependent, avoidant and obsessive-compulsive. Each has their own twists and nuances and can be personified into caricatures – suspicious, worried, angry – a bit like the seven dwarves.

Each day, out and about, I see displays of histrionics, antisociality, avoidance, narcissism. I spot them in my friends and family and have them pointed out in myself. But does this mean we will all come to the attention of mental health services? Course not. Personality disorder becomes pathological when the intensity of these characteristics cannot be regulated, and the person 'acts out' repeatedly in ways that are harmful and risky. These are the patients who come to our attention. These are the Bobbys.

There have been literary and cinematic attempts to depict personality disorders (think of Glenn Close's character in *Fatal Attraction*, a brilliant portrayal of a borderline personality type; or Gordon Gecko in *Wall Street*, a purity of the corporate asocial type). Shocking though it is to admit, we feel we know these characters, recognise the traits.

Today, someone with a personality disorder may be offered a combination of medication and/or specialist psychological input. This may be as dialectical behavioural therapy, created by American psychologist Marsha Linehan, whose approach combines traditional cognitive theory with techniques of mindfulness and acceptance.

Among mental health professionals, working with patients with personality disorder is like Marmite. Some are drawn to the social aspects of the job, for often this client group has housing, drug, alcohol or criminal justice related issues; some like working with risk, building relationships with people who've been trampled on and are mistrustful, and unpredictable.

But others in my profession bear an ardent dislike for those with these diagnoses. They don't believe they are real mental disorders, and consider them to be frustrating time-wasters. Words like selfish and manipulative get bandied about to describe these 'raging PDs'; out of hours, over a few drinks, the slurs can really spill out.

I suspect I know where this kind of cynicism originates. Moreso than any other client group, personality disorder patients can be consuming, anxiety provoking, gruelling.

At times, I've felt I've been getting somewhere with Bobby – building rapport that will mean she doesn't need to publicly hurt herself to get the attention she craves – but her capacity for temperance, regulation, and her ability to make and commit to wise choices will change like the British weather. Before long, she does something – self-harming, overdosing, threating to jump off a bridge – or in this case, putting herself in the traffic.

It can feel deliberate, aimed at me.

I was asked to work with Bobby six months prior.

'I've got an interesting case for you,' my manager says, almost looking at me. 'You may've heard of her.'

'Oh, right,' I say, removing my bike helmet, nodding. 'I know the name, I think.'

Course I've heard of Bobby. Everyone has.

Her referral came to the team via her GP, a physician at his wits' end. Bobby was pestering him for sedatives, sick notes, threatening suicide in the reception when she felt unheard. Over the years she'd been given diagnoses ranging from anxiety, depression, poly-substance dependency, attention deficit hyperactivity disorder, and, perhaps most tellingly, emotionally unstable personality disorder, previously known as borderline. It was agreed, much to Bobby's approval, that a specialist mental health team was needed to meet her complex needs.

By now, I'm one of the more experienced members of the team, used to working with the risky, oppositional patients. Bobby would be a challenge. I was game.

'OK,' I say. 'I'll try.'

Somehow, before I've even contacted Bobby, she's discovered the name of her new care coordinator and begins calling the team, wanting to speak to me. She's also figured out my NHS email address, and a list of messages clogs up my inbox, asking for a time and date of our first appointment.

This gets my back up: it's normally me tracking the patients, not the other way round.

Before replying, I look at her medical notes. They read like a Ken Loach script. Alcoholic mum. Non-existent dad. Foster care. Bullying. Teenage abortions. Petty crime. Substance abuse. Suicide attempts.

She's had stints in rehab, prison, crisis houses, refuges, and has been admitted multiple times to hospital, all with little demonstrative impact. Her offending history lists five pages of petty offences ranging from shoplifting, public disorder and, most commonly, wasting police time.

In the past month she's been picked up at train tracks and bridges as far north as Morecambe, as far south as Beachy Head. Each of her three previous care coordinators gives the same weary headshake and offers a similar version of events: at first they were flavour of the month, bombarded with calls and emails. Then they made a minor error, unforgivable in Bobby's eyes. In response, she ramped up the self-harm and suicide threats.

'Any advice?' I ask.

'Be careful,' each says, as if I'm a gladiator entering an amphitheatre.

I go in prepared. And during that first meeting with Bobby, which takes place at the community mental health team base, I figure I can handle her – OK, she's blunt, direct, loquacious, with an off-kilter sense of humour and zero filter. She remarks on my spots, my Harry Potter specs, my wedding ring, probing, trying to get a rise; when that doesn't work, she mentions berating her elderly neighbour that morning to the point of tears, kicking an errant cat, and she repeatedly shows her self-harm wounds on her arms like medals of honour, all with the intention of triggering me. But I stay straight-faced. There's nothing insurmountable. Not yet.

'You like your job?' she says, cracking open a Coke can.

'Yes,' I say.

'Why?'

'I get to meet people from all walks of life and try to help them.' A pause. 'Do you like your job?' Bobby works Saturdays at Nags' Head Market, Islington, flogging moody perfumes and fake designer handbags.

'Yeah,' she says. 'I get to meet people from all walks of life too. We're kinda similar aren't we, El? I reckon we're going to get on.'

I smile.

'So what're you planning? How will you get me well?'

'What does "get me well" mean?'

'I want to stop thinking about killing myself all the time.'

'OK. What else?'

'I want to stop going to A&E and getting in trouble with the police.'

'That's good. What else?'

She thinks. 'I want to enjoy life. Have friends. Relationships.'

I'm impressed – she seems motivated. When I smile again, she smiles back, and chugs on her Coke.

'My job is to support you towards those goals,' I say.

'Instead of taking yourself to A&E and self-harming, I want you to use me. To offload with. But to do that, we need to have an agreement, Bobby.'

She nods keenly.

'We'll meet here once a week to discuss what's going on for you. And we can have no more than two ten-minute phone calls outside of that meeting. These will be your limit.'

'Why not more?'

'Because I have other patients to see. That's more than they get.'

'But I'm more complex than them.'

'Says who?'

She thinks some more. 'Who will I call if I'm struggling at night or the weekend?'

'There are crisis lines. There're organisations like the Samaritans too. And there are the distraction techniques you've been introduced to.'

These techniques are sensory, and for some, effective – elastic bands to snap against her skin, 'safe songs' to transcend, calming oils and perfumes to sniff like analgesics – all used to pull Bobby away from that visceral need to hurt herself.

'But in the long term,' I add, 'you won't need to reach out for help when you're struggling. Right?'

She makes a sour face, as if she's bitten down on a mouldy lemon.

'We're going to work on ways for you to manage those intense feelings better. Emotional regulation. Grounding. Resilience.'

She drinks from the can slowly, ponderously, and purses

her lips into a frown. 'You're different to the other care coordinators I've had.'

'How?'

'You're tougher.'

Smiling, I say, 'I'm just being straight with you, Bobby. I want to be realistic about what I can and cannot do.'

The frown turns razor-tight. Time passes, and she nods. 'OK. I'll do what you say.' And I think, for a moment, that I've got somewhere.

'Ten a.m. sharp. Tuesday mornings,' I say. 'We can talk Monday and Friday on the phone. No calls, emails or turning up unannounced. And under no circumstances are you to contact emergency services or take yourself to A&E unless you're dying. Can you do it, Bobby? Do we have a deal?'

'Deal,' she says, swirling the last of her Coke down. 'Talk Friday.'

She heads for the door, leaving her Coke can on the floor, perhaps by mistake, but I suspect as a calling card, to remember her while she's gone.

To be fair to Bobby, she really does try at first, attending our appointments as agreed, limiting the calls and emails, not crashing up at A&E. When we meet, I'm taken by her quirky imagination, her quickdraw quips, her willingness to try new vocations I suggest – animal care, going to the gym, mindfulness apps – ways to placate her thoughts. I wonder if I might be making a breakthrough.

For my part I maintain boundaries, not missing our meetings or calls, never deviating from what's been agreed. I want to show her that if I say I'll do something I won't let her down; by the same token I expect the same. It seems to work, the structure providing a segue into meaningful conversation.

'I don't like the term personality disorder,' she says a few weeks in. 'Sounds like there's people out there who have an ordered personality. You got one of those, El?'

I tell her I don't, but we're not here to talk about me, and she gives a wry laugh.

Bobby is without question a textbook PD patient – dependent, defiant, needy, avoidant, with a list of abnormal coping strategies, self-harm being the most prolific, which we soon talk about freely.

'I dunno why I cut,' she says, rolling up a sleeve. 'It's not to kill myself.'

'What's going through your head when it happens?' I say.

She thinks a moment. 'Nothin'. That's just it. I feel dead a lot of the time. Hurting myself, seeing the blood, it helps me feel alive. You know?'

I nod. 'Keep talking. See where it goes.'

Bobby thinks. 'Rather than just have the emptiness, I cut myself to feel full. But it never lasts. After, I look at what I did to myself and I feel ashamed.' She drinks from her Coke can. 'I haven't cut myself in three weeks, El. That's long for me. I want to get better.'

I believe her.

She places the can on the floor and leaves. Right then, I feel admiration for Bobby.

A few weeks later, when things turn, I try to remember today.

*

My mistake is to take a week of annual leave without due consideration for Bobby. Hardly a capital crime, but to her, it was a big wrongy.

Clare, Spencer and I journey to Lancashire, Clare's home turf, to scout possible areas to move to in the not-too-distant future. The past few months we've been mulling over the idea of relocating, seeking a bigger home and a calmer life, where the cost of living can be matched by a nurse's salary. What should've been a relaxing jaunt turns into a migraine. On day two, while we're walking along the Fylde coast, my Facebook feed starts pinging with scores of messages. When I look at the sender, the profile picture is a Coke can.

ANSWER YOUR PHONE!

REPLY TO EMAILS!

HELP ME!!!

Many mental health professionals hide their social media identities with pseudonyms – now I know why. With a sinking feeling I retrieve my work phone from the car. Turning it on, I find over a hundred missed calls, texts and emails from Bobby. All say pretty much the same thing: she's unhappy with the colleague I asked to sub for me, doesn't feel heard and is thinking about doing something because I've let her down.

I try to ignore this threat, uphold boundaries, remind myself that I'm not Bobby's dad – she's a grown woman, and she needs to learn that she cannot behave like this whenever she doesn't feel validated. But when her messages turn nasty – accusing me of being unprofessional, blaming me for her impending death – I cave and ring her. She answers immediately, as if she's poised by the phone.

'You never thought about me!' she blurts.

'I did,' I say. 'I arranged for my colleague to check in with you.'

'She's rubbish! I only got a six-minute call! Not ten!'

I can't believe what I'm hearing. When I try and say as much, Bobby explodes. For the next minute I hold the phone away from my ear as she bawls and curses. When she's calmed enough to come in, I say, 'Bobby, I'm back next week. I'm going now.'

'If I die it's because of you.'

I squeeze the handset.

'Well?'

'Bye,' I say, and hang up.

When she tries calling back immediately, I turn the phone off.

'Everything OK?' Clare says, she and Spencer staring at me expectantly.

'It's fine,' I say through gritted teeth, and determine to put this out of my mind.

When I return to work the following Monday, Bobby is still alive. But she's in hospital.

It transpires that after our call she took herself to A&E, lacerating her forearm with a torn-up Coke tin in front of staff, enough to require stitches. When I go and see her, she's ensconced in a bay on a ward. Her right arm is bandaged. Seeing me, she says, 'Hey, how was your holiday?'

'Bobby,' I say, 'we need to talk about what you did.'

She looks perplexed.

'You can't contact me privately, ever. Finding me on

Facebook – it's not OK. And it's not what we agreed.'

'We agreed that you'd meet me once a week and give me two calls, ten minutes. That woman you had covering didn't do that.'

'You can't be serious.'

Bobby smiles gleefully. She is serious. She's enjoying this too.

A nasty ick forms in my gut. I try to remember that human side I'd seen in Bobby, her vulnerability; but right then I don't like the woman, and I don't want to be around her one bit. Admitting this doesn't feel great. In fact, it feels mean. I got into this line of work because I'm interested in people and want to help them. I never envisioned having an aversion like this.

I've learned that these responses aren't uncommon. The Freudians call it countertransference – the emotions, biases, prejudices and general baggage brought up from being in the presence of someone else. I've had instances where countertransference is helpful in gauging where someone is at, sensing that even though they're saying, 'Of course I'm happy', everything in their manner screams, 'No, I'm not!'

With Bobby, it's a blocker. In the weeks that follow, I find being around her generates feelings in me that go from moderate to pounding, so much so that at times I can barely tolerate being in her company. During another Tuesday meeting, it becomes apparent that she isn't blind to this.

'You don't like me much,' she says.

I fake affront. 'You're my patient,' I reply. 'I don't like or dislike y—'

'Yeah, you don't like me. After I contacted you on holiday.

You're probably planning on discharging me. But that's OK. I forgive you.'

'What?'

She nods. 'And when I'm dead and buried, and you're feeling guilty, wondering if there was more you could've done, remember that.'

I stare at her and she stares at me and neither of us says a thing.

Bobby, who has recently dyed her buzz cut a lurid orange, and wears a silver hoop piercing through her septum, looks bright, colourful. But her eyes jar with the rest of her countenance; dull, shuttered, languorous eyes, the irises pale blue, the pupils ink black, and with no expression at all, seeming to see me and see through me too, as if I'm made of glass.

She's right, of course – I am planning to discharge her, and have been working on it for weeks. I've been her longest-running care coordinator, which is an achievement. We made some inroads in that time too, plugging her into various pursuits, skilling her up with some coping strategies. But now we've arrived at an impasse. It seems a good time to step back.

What proves the obstacle is Bobby's ability to sabotage my efforts. When I begin broaching the subject the following week, she makes it clear that if I do discharge her, there's a fair-to-middling chance she won't be here.

'Why?' I say. 'Why do you want to stay with my team? What am I offering you?'

She shakes her head. 'You can't just leave me.'

'I don't understand.'

'I'm ill.'

'I don't think I'm any use though, Bobby.'

'If something happens, it'll be on you.'

'Stop saying that. It's blackmail.'

She drinks the last swig from her Coke can. Then she crumples it and gazes at the jagged edges of tin.

She's messing with my head, trying to uncoil anxiety, lead me into a dark web of fear. It's working too. Our meetings have gone from constructive, with boundaries, to uncomfortable, passive aggressive. I feel like I'm slipping into a quagmire.

'OK.' She stands up. 'So we'll park the discharge idea. Speak to you on Friday?'

I nod.

She leaves the room, her crumpled Coke can left on the floor, this time not a reminder of her existence, but like a declaration of war.

We carry on, meeting weekly at my community base and having our two phone calls. There's no progress, and no crises. Just strained conversations and stretched silences.

The routine changes when Bobby needs a favour. Her Personal Independent Payment benefit is due for review and she goes into a nosedive, seeing it as a vendetta against her. Seeing this as the first tangible bit of support I can give Bobby, I offer to accompany her to the appeal meeting and advocate on her behalf.

When we arrive at the centre, a dreary Social Services building with steel benches mounted to the floor and 'Violence Will Not Be Tolerated' posters everywhere, we're informed the assessor is sick and the meeting will need to be rescheduled. Bobby is incandescent. She points a dagger finger at the receptionist, tells her if something happens to her, it's on them. Then she crumbles to the floor like a rag doll and starts wailing and cursing.

'Fucking bastards! Fuck, shit!'

The other customers stare. The receptionist looks at me with a frown. It's the same frown I've had when Spencer has a meltdown in public.

'Come on, Bobby,' I say, crouching down.

She stays put, hammering the floor.

'Why me? Why fucking me!'

The receptionist radios Security. Moments later, a wiry African gent in a flat cap arrives. Seeing him, Bobby suggests he perform a sex act on himself.

Aware this is escalating, I scoop Bobby up, make my apologies, usher us to the door. Foul of mood, she thunders from the complex just as the skies open into a torrential storm. I scamper to keep up. Before long we're both soaked. But the rain appears to have tempered the storm in Bobby enough for me to speak to her.

'Sorry,' she says, stopping, looking at me. The rain has washed away her tears.

I nod.

'You're all wet.'

'It's fine,' I say, as raindrops careen down my nose and eyelids.

'I live over there,' she says. 'Come back till the rain's stopped.'

I hesitate. As a community mental health nurse, I often do

home visits, alone. But I've never wanted to for Bobby. The prospect of going to her home now doesn't thrill me. But the rain isn't abating. And it dawns on me that this is the most meaningful our conversation has been in weeks. So I go.

'I'll stick the kettle on,' she says as soon as we're inside her local authority home. 'What do you think of my gaff?'

'Nice,' I lie, removing my drenched coat, taking it in.

It's dark, spare, a boxy studio with a kitchenette and bathroom. There's little in the way of furniture or décor. A few plastic apples and oranges in a bowl, a bunch of fake roses in a vase; the sofa, which makes do as a bed, is faux leather, torn, taped up, positioned to partially hide the scuds and holes in the stud wall; plug-in diffusers blast out strawberry fumes to mask the stagnant mould that cloys; family photos adorn the walls, sepia images of happy couples with happy kids, all holding hands on beaches and promenades.

'Who's in the photos?' I say.

'Dunno,' Bobby says. 'I bought them from charity shops.'

'You mean you don't know who these people are?'

'Yeah.'

'So why hang them up?'

Bobby thinks; the rain rattles against the window. 'To feel normal.'

Carefully, I say, 'What does that mean?'

'You're normal. You've got a missus at home, right? A kid? A nice place to live?'

'Just because I have those things, doesn't mean I'm normal.'

'I bet you don't go around doing stuff like this?' She rolls up her sleeve, flashes her latest cuts and burns, fresh, angry-looking. 'Huh?'

A change befalls her then. Her face remains passive, her stare unwavering. But her eyes leak again. Tears run from her while the rest of her is still. These aren't crocodile tears, and they're not a resurgence from her tantrum earlier. I'm seeing a fleeting glimpse of Bobby. My ick crumbles away.

We stand like this together until the kettle clicks off and she makes us a brew.

Maybe, I reason, my presence in her life is having a benefit, helping in ways I haven't considered. I haven't abandoned her, despite her efforts; I won't let her down the way so many have. A part of Bobby is daring to trust, but another part of her is pulling away, telling her I'm a cretin, a liar, and, eventually, I'll let her down too.

It's this, I'm sure, that triggers what happens next.

Most mental health professionals have been sacked by a patient. It happens for all kinds of reasons: sometimes the patient feels abandoned; sometimes they take offence at a term or phrase used; sometimes we make a mistake or put our foot in it; sometimes it's a simple personality clash; and sometimes it's a mystery.

It can feel strange, abrupt, unexpected, even a relief.

With Bobby, I'm taken wholly by surprise. On a frosty December morning, while cycling to work to meet her for our weekly face-to-face, the front wheel of my bike skids on some black ice at the mouth of a junction. Suddenly, from upright and pedalling, I'm supine, staring skyward, my chest panting, my left knee numb.

Cursing, I get up, begin wheeling my bike to the kerb-side. I make it about ten feet, then wince. My whole body starts trembling, and the numbness leaves my knee, replaced with a pulsating pain.

I one-eighty, wheeling my bike home. Twenty minutes later I arrive home, ready to collapse. Clutching a pack of frozen peas on my knee, I text my manager, explain that I can't come in. Then I gobble some co-dydramol from the cupboard, collapse on the sofa, and shut my eyes.

What I neglect to do is alert Bobby. My bad.

While I'm sleeping, Bobby arrives at the office expecting me. Instead, I'm a no-show. The news that I'm off sick has failed to reach the receptionist at the front desk, and she can only apologise to Bobby and suggest there's been a mistake. But in Bobby's mind this validates a suspicion she's had all along. I'm bad. I'll let her down. Like everyone lets her down.

When I come to, it's lunchtime. My knee is like an overripe peach and I've got an ugly feeling in my tummy that something bad has happened. I switch on my phone, see the texts from Bobby. It's like a boulder plunging into a lake.

I call her, and the barrage begins:

'Who do you think you are, mucking me about, leaving me stood there like a div? I've a good mind to—'

'Whoa,' I interject. 'It was an accident, Bobby. Don't overreact.'

'Fuck you!'

Now, on top of shock, I'm angry. 'I didn't mean to fall off my bike. It wasn't aimed at you. Calm down.'

She doesn't calm down. Her rage is more intense than the pain in my knee.

'Let's reschedule,' I say.

A pregnant pause.

'Bobby?'

Nothing.

'I'm sorry. I'll be back to work the day after tomorrow. Come in and see me then.'

She hangs up, and I look at the ceiling. The rasp of her screaming echoes in my ears. But behind the anger I hear a girl afraid.

Bobby doesn't turn up to see me. When I try calling, my number has been blocked. There's no response from texts or emails either. She's gone.

I figure she's angry, giving me a taste of my own medicine. Fair enough.

But within a few days there's still nothing and I'm starting to worry. I consider going to her flat, a cold call. She could've hurt herself badly. Self-harmers are known to lacerate arteries by mistake. She could need help.

In the end, I don't.

'Doing that will just reinforce her dependency,' a colleague says. 'She'll be back,' says another.

They're right.

The following Monday, I'm called to a meeting. I'm expecting the worst: Bobby's been found dead. But that's not the case. She's alive, well, and royally pissed off. She's posted a complaint about me, listing all my failures, my inability to support her, my mean, cruel attitude and her wish to never see me again.

'Jesus Christ,' I say.

An investigation is required, a formality my manager assures me, whereby I'm interviewed about these allegations to determine whether there is any meat on the bone.

Nothing she's complained about can be substantiated. But the fact that she went to the trouble of writing this letter hurts me.

'Told you to be careful with her,' someone in the office says.

'Yes,' I say.

'Bet you're relieved you can discharge her now?'

'Yes.'

In truth, I have an emptiness in me too, maybe a small taste of what Bobby experiences daily.

'She's been arrested?' I say to the gravelly sergeant on the end of the phone. 'What for?'

'Public disturbance,' he says, 'racism, criminal damage and wasting police time. The list goes on.'

'What happened?'

'She walked into a hospital A&E, started cutting her arm. When the staff tried to move her on, she became abusive. Ended up walloping a care assistant. Hurling racist abuse.'

'Oh dear.'

'She may well get a custodial for this. We interviewed her under caution. And now she's started headbanging in her cell. Says she's going to kill herself.'

'Yes,' I say, 'that sounds like Bobby.'

He clears his throat. 'She's asked to see you.'

I take a deep breath.

And so I get back on my bike and pedal off to Islington, where Bobby is being held at the local police station. I flash my ID to the desk clerk, get shown through several secure doors and walk into a custody area.

WE DON'T USE WORDS LIKE 'CRAZY'

A stern-looking sergeant sits at a desk, punching buttons on his keyboard. When I say who I am, he stares at me as if this is all my fault.

'You from the mental health?'

I tell him I am.

Two things are apparent about this sergeant: the first, he owns the gravelly voice on the phone; the second, he doesn't much like Bobby, his job or me, it would seem.

'What can you tell me, sergeant?'

He starts reading from her rap sheet. Since Bobby sacked me, she's gone on a downward spiral – shoplifting, drugs, fraternising with undesirables, presenting at A&E and her GP surgery, threatening suicide, coming close a few times.

'What's wrong with her?' the sergeant says. 'I mean, why'd someone go and do all that?'

'She's diagnosed with personality disorder,' I say.

'What's that?'

'It's a mental illness.'

Either he's got a bad case of hay fever or that's a snort of derision. 'Don't get me wrong, I'm sympathetic,' he says, with all the compassion of a pickaxe, 'but she's a real drain, this woman. My officers, they should be out catching burglars and pickpockets. Sometimes we run out of patience with these people.'

These people. The words hang.

He takes me through doors, more doors, and towards the cells. Keys rattle, doors clank, and a moment later I'm stood in the doorway of a gloomy cell, looking at Bobby crouched down in a squat against the wall.

She's changed her appearance again – her hair lurid green; her ears, lips and face a trove of piercings. She's lost weight; her Under Armour trackie is now baggy and she looks like a child in grown-up clothing. Even in the dark I can make out a large yellowing bruise around her right temple where she's been headbanging, and cuts, scuds, burns and scratches over her neck and hands.

'Hi,' I say.

She stares up with flat, dead eyes.

'How're you doing, Bobby?'

She laughs; a sharp, mirthless laugh. 'Fuck off.'

I turn, doing as she says.

'Where are you going?'

I look back. 'I'm fucking off.'

Her bottom lip quivers. 'They want to charge me.'

'Yes.'

'I could go to prison.'

'You could.'

'You can get me off, El. Tell them it's not my fault. Explain about my mental health—'

'They know about that, Bobby.'

'But you can tell it better. You can explain how—'

'No.'

She flinches; her eyes fill up. 'This is your fault.'

'I'm sorry, Bobby, I don't think it is.'

'I'm ill, and you abandoned me.' Her voice echoes off the enclosed space. 'Well,' she says, 'what are you going to do?'

I shake my head.

'If I kill myself, it's on you.'

She stares and stares until the anger bleeds from her eyes

and then she squeezes her eyelids shut and brings her palms to her face.

'Fuck off,' she says.

This time I do.

I thank the sergeant, buy a few cans of Coke from a vending machine in the waiting area, ask that he give them to Bobby when she's calmer, make sure she doesn't lacerate herself with them. Then I leave.

Outside it's dark. The moon hangs like a pendulum in the coal-black night.

I'm tired. My breath appears in plumes. My head is cauliflower cheese. For a few minutes I traipse about, unable to find where I secured my bike. When, finally, I locate the rack, my trusty two-wheeler is gone. All that's left is my D-lock that's been cut through with an angle-grinder left on the pavement like a pile of ribs.

I consider going back to the police station, reporting a theft. But at that moment I haven't got the mental health for it, or any of it.

Instead, I start walking.

Back to my normal life.

That Joke Isn't Funny Anymore

'Why didn't you just section Dan?' the coroner says, staring at me querulously over her specs. 'If you were concerned, you should've got him into hospital, and we wouldn't be here now.'

Within the square dock of the inquest courtroom my toes curl and my knuckles clench.

'It wasn't that simple,' I say, glancing at the dozen attendants, which includes Simone – the hamster cheeks and emerald eyes a match for her late twin brother. 'I was concerned he'd make an attempt, but I had no idea when he'd do it. You can't admit someone forever.'

'But he was mentally ill?' There's incredulity in the coroner's voice that grates.

'He was diagnosed with depression, yes.'

'He'd stated plans to end his life?'

'At some point. Like I said, he wasn't specific.'

'He had ways and means to follow through on the threat?'

'Yes.'

'And he was a single male who used to be a mental health nurse, I gather. A high-risk demographic group.'

I nod.

She makes an exasperated sound, like she has a trapped disc. 'Surely there's more you could've done, Mr Sweeney?'

Surely.

Three months prior, I was asked to work with Dan.

It's been a tough year. The legacy of Brexit, austerity cuts, the abolition of trainee bursaries all lead to gaping wounds in services that slowly bleed out, causing a feeling of panic and a malaise among those of us who work in the trenches.

My caseload has swollen to the high thirties, an impossible number to manage; instead, firefighting seems the appropriate analogy. For each patient, we're expected to complete vast, repetitious amounts of admin: support plans, risk assessments, itemising each moment of the day on complex spreadsheets. Because of this, I can see patients twice, maybe three times a month at best, to assess their mental state. Outside of this I have no idea how they are. It feels unsafe.

Managers acknowledge these shortfalls and insist they have our backs if the you-know-what hits the fan. Yet if something does go wrong, it is invariably the lowly nurse hauled in for answers. That's how it seems to go in the NHS. The aforementioned you-know-what rolls down.

Of course, there've been staff walk-outs, colleagues throwing in the towel and being replaced by new faces, enthusiastic at first, but, by week two, lethargic, disgruntled, dismayed. There's been a swathe of stress-related sicknesses on my team, colleagues crying, popping antidepressants, chuffing cigarettes, gorging cream cakes, guzzling booze as an outlet.

If we were working in a more salubrious setting, things might feel more tolerable. But the office is a decaying asbestos-ridden state with one toilet, regularly clogged. Radiators are cranked up to full blast all year, meaning in the summer we're forced to wedge windows open and haul in industrial fans. And they wonder why the NHS is in such a financial pickle.

Amid it all comes Dan.

On paper, he's a straightforward case – a single man struggling with low mood and suicidal ideation. Bread and butter to me. Then I delve deeper, and my curiosity is piqued: like me, Dan is approaching forty; he was born and raised in northeast London; and, most significantly, for ten years he worked as a mental health nurse.

'Don't end up like me,' he says the first time we meet, sitting opposite each other at a Costa coffee shop in Camden.

'Like you?'

He drinks from his cappuccino, the chocolate leaving a brown moustache below his nose as he lowers the mug. 'Joyless,' he says, and gives me a wink.

Meeting here was Dan's idea. It's busy, brimming with the echelons of London: advertising execs and hedge fund investors stir coffees alongside homeless folk and addicts waiting to jack up in the loo. Dan seems to like the diversity, being around people.

'I miss doing your job,' he says, 'but I could never go back to it.'

'Why not?'

'Because it draws you in, then chews you up. People say you can't catch mental illness the way you catch a cold. But you can. Ever heard that saying? You go into a barber shop enough times—'

'You'll come out with a haircut,' I say.

We laugh.

There's a James Corden quality to Dan, with the puffy cheeks, the chappy grin, the sparkly emerald eyes, the clownishness; he's the kind of guy you could airlift into a cocktail party or a working men's club and not have to worry. A big lad, he favours Gap T-shirts, loose jeans, DM 8-holes, and is never without a flat cap; he's got this earthy laugh that he uses plentifully, and which seems to light him from the inside.

Yet there's a sadness to Dan too, of the quiet, profound kind. I hear it in the absences between his words, when his laughter ends abruptly; he darkens, and his eyes flit away from mine and seem to zero in on nothing.

He quit mental health nursing following his first lengthy stay in hospital. In the preceding months, he'd lapsed into a state of depression, the fifth episode in his life, which culminated in a serious overdose at the end of a nightshift. His entry into the profession, he goes on to tell me, came from experiences as a kid. Bullied at school, neglected by his parents, he dragged a ball and chain of issues into adulthood, and like so many mental health professionals, he figured working in the field would fix him.

For a while, it did.

Then it didn't, and things fell apart.

At the time, he'd been working as a staff nurse in a

revered south London mental health unit; he was good at his job, well respected, always the first to volunteer and go that extra mile...

But those miles chipped away. Now he's unemployed. Medicated to the teeth. He's had the alphabet of treatments: Cognitive Behavioural Therapy (CBT), Eye Movement Desensitization and Reprocessing (EMDR), Electroconvulsive Therapy (ECT), Trans-Cranial Magnetic Therapy (TMS); he's had psychodynamic psychotherapy, psychedelic drug therapy, Gestalt therapy, primal scream treatment.

And he remains joyless.

'What do you reckon is wrong with me?' he says, leaning in.

I search for an answer, a tried response from my toolkit. But Dan isn't a typical patient. He's savvy from years on the job, with a well-tuned bullshit detector. He's read the same books I have, had the same tricky exchanges with patients, been asked the same questions.

'I don't know,' I eventually say. 'What do you reckon?'

'Chicken and egg,' he says.

I tilt my head.

'What came first? If I hadn't had problems, I wouldn't have got into mental health nursing. But if I hadn't been a mental health nurse, my problems wouldn't have got to this stage. Surrounded by misery and trauma every day – it gets into your bones. I mean, it's not normal. Talking about death and self-harm, day in, day out. You think you're desensitised. But it seeps through the cracks and darkens your soul. And then, when you're not looking...' He brings his fist into his other hand. Then he laughs haughtily.

I try to laugh too, but it comes as a hacking cough. What Dan's just said is a bone in my windpipe.

'I shouldn't be saying all this to you,' he says. 'You seem a nice guy. It's going to wreck your head, isn't it?'

'It's OK,' I say, adding, 'you're not the first person I've met who's talked like this.'

But he's the first ex-mental health nurse who has.

'So what's the secret?' I say. 'How do I—'

'How do you keep from turning into me?' He grins. 'Christ knows. Do yoga. Go vegan. Find God. Take drugs. But get an outlet. Some joy in your life. Understand?'

We finish our coffees. As we're standing, pulling on our coats, he says fondly, inconsequentially, 'You know I'll do it.'

I look at him quizzically.

'You know what I mean.'

I've had patients threaten suicide before. But with Dan it feels different. Not said as a threat, or in desperation. It's his conviviality that bothers me.

'I *do* know what you mean,' I say. 'But why are you telling me this? What do you expect me to do with the information?'

'To be prepared.'

I shake my head. 'If you're so certain, why do all this? Coming to meet me, to chat? There must be a bit of hope. If not, why not just get on with it?'

Dan thinks on this a long time. 'I like you,' he says. 'You remind me of me.'

'Then I need you to keep a bit of faith that things can get better. Don't put me in a bind.'

He shrugs.

'What about your family? Haven't you got parents? You mentioned a twin sister? Won't they miss you?'

'Trying to find protective factors, right?' He grins. 'Look, I'm not saying I'm about to leave this coffee shop and jump in front of a lorry. Right now, talking to you, I'm OK.'

'There you go,' I say. 'You've got to remember th—'

'But I know me,' he cuts in. 'I know where I'm headed. From one nurse to another. OK?'

I'm flummoxed. Is he joking? Mucking about? 'But how can you be so sure?' I say. 'I refuse to believe there's not more that can be done to help you.'

At this, Dan's eyes retract into that fog of inwardness. 'There's nothing more. Remember, I know all the tricks in the book.'

Now anger pinches me as well as confusion. I refuse to believe that Dan's fate is a foregone conclusion. All right, he worked in mental health, knows about the treatments, the pills, the talking therapies, yada yada. But it can't be the case that all avenues are exhausted, and Dan's just a ticking bomb.

Can it?

A month or so before his death, there's an escalation.

We meet at Costa and he's on crutches, his right ankle in a cast.

I enquire why, and his lips purse. 'It was my birthday. Forty. I had a couple of gins, and I felt maudlin. Anyway, one thing led to another and I climbed on the kitchen table and fell. I guess it wasn't built for people my size.'

'Jesus,' I say, feeling my face turn aghast. 'What were you

doing on the table?' I want him to say he'd been changing a lightbulb or singing karaoke.

He shrugs. 'Experimenting.'

'Experimenting?'

He's serious, and I'm shocked – by what took place and by his cheeriness.

'Are you going to do it again?' I ask. 'Experimenting, I mean?'

'No.' He points at his ankle cast. 'I can't, can I? Not when I'm in this. And I've ruined a perfectly good table too.'

I stare, and he stares back, and then he explodes into laughter. Without meaning to, I laugh with him, but it's an uncomfortable laugh, the kind that comes after a sick joke.

'Belated happy birthday,' I say.

'Cheers,' Dan says, wiping his eyes. 'What date's yours?'

I tell him.

'Don't do what I did when you turn the big four-oh.'

'Don't worry.'

'And promise me you'll laugh about this afterwards. That you'll remember me this way.'

To my shame, I say that I will.

That afternoon, I ask my team psychiatrist to offer Dan an appointment to assess his mental state. She moves around her clinic, and it takes place the following morning at the team base.

Afterwards, as Dan hobbles from the site on crutches, the psychiatrist, a young, capable registrar, comes and sits with me at my desk and holds up her hands in befuddlement.

'He doesn't seem a risk to himself now,' she says.

I nod.

'He doesn't seem particularly depressed either.'

I nod again.

'He just seems . . .' She removes her hipster glasses, stares up, struggling for the word.

'Joyless?' I suggest.

She nods.

Henceforth, I discuss Dan in team meetings, wanting to get others' impressions, see if they have ideas. Some colleagues think he must be psychotic and should be sectioned to hospital. Some think I should discharge him as there's no role for me. No one knows quite what to do for certain. Including me.

I scratch my head. I mull. I get angry. Worried. Sad.

At my wits' end, I present his case to our Trust's high-risk panel, a forum to discuss particularly concerning patients. The panel consists of three seniors – a clinical director, a psychotherapist and a consultant psychiatrist – who sit in a horseshoe and give advice.

After explaining Dan's case, outlining what's been tried and the fact that he's still cheerfully talking of his impending death, the trio look at each other and back at me and sigh collectively.

'You think he's going to complete a suicide then?' the pinstriped clinical director says, his voice imbued with plummy authority.

'Yes,' I say.

'You just don't know how, or when, or what to do?'

'Correct.'

'Tricky.'

I wait for more.

'Existential crisis,' the psychotherapist says, her sensible grey voice matching her sensible grey suit. 'People who've worked in this sector are often the toughest to help.'

'OK,' I say, my nails digging into my palms, 'but have you got any tips?'

'Keep meeting him regularly,' the psychiatrist offers, stroking his Dumbledore beard. 'Have frank conversations about life and death. You could suggest he read some Durkheim and Camus. Try to get him to open up.'

'I do all those things,' I say. 'He is open with me. Very open. It doesn't seem to help. Anything else?'

'Make sure your notes are up to date,' the clinical director adds. 'In case anything does happen.'

When I tell Dan of this meeting, he bursts into giggles.

'Read Durkheim and Camus. Bloody genius!'

For a moment I want to laugh with him, share some gallows humour with a fellow nurse about a patient...

Then I remember the patient is Dan.

You'd have thought I'd be prepped, but news of Dan's death is like a stylus needle abruptly scratched across a vinyl record.

I arrive at work on Monday morning. My manager and her service head are in a side office. They call me in and tell me frankly.

'His twin sister went to his flat,' the service head says. 'He'd left a note pinned to the door saying not to come in under any circumstances but to call the ambulance and police.'

'What did she do?' I say.

'She went in. Found him hanging from the kitchen ceiling.

Stone-cold. He'd done his research since last time. Found out about ligaturing. Knew how to do it right.'

There's a beating silence.

'Are you OK?' my manager says.

I nod. The world has tilted.

'There'll be an autopsy. Then an inquest. We'll have to submit a serious incident report too. But don't worry about any of that.'

'OK.'

'I don't think you could've done any more.'

'Yes,' I say, although the words whistle through me. I head for the door.

'You did update his notes, though,' the service head says. I turn and stare. 'Didn't you?'

I *did* update Dan's notes, many times, and a fat lot of good that did.

That night I have a nightmare, about ligatures tied to kitchen ceilings and sisters finding brothers dead. I wake up panting and sweating, a train screeching through my skull. The following day I call in sick and stay home, hugging a pillow, watching daytime TV with the sound down. I plan to get back to work the next day, but something in me seems to have stopped working.

Instead, I take another day off, then another, lounging in my dressing gown, eating breakfast cereals from the box, making cups of tea and not drinking them, reading books and giving up after a few pages.

I don't believe there was any more I could've done to save Dan. Sectioning him wasn't the answer. Even if he had been detained in hospital they wouldn't have been able to treat him. At some point he would've come out. And then he'd have done it.

So why am I cut up? I hadn't known Dan more than a few months. I'd never seen his home, met his family. He wasn't a mate. He was a patient. What's wrong?

Simple. He was a mental nurse. Like me.

I take a week of leave. On a whim, I book onto a writing retreat in Hebden Bridge, West Yorkshire.

Creative writing is a hobby I've been dabbling with for years, splurging ideas onto the page, seeing where they go. I'm pleasantly surprised that I can string sentences together and find doing so strangely cathartic. My output is mostly rambling, metaphysical vignettes, noir poetry-prose and adolescent pyrotechnics with supernatural goings-on.

Once, I'd shared a few of my ideas with Dan, knowing he liked to read.

Flatly, he dismantled each and told me why. 'You need something real to write about. Not this Stephen King imitation bollocks.'

'Any ideas?'

'Write about the job.'

The job.

The week at the retreat is ideal. I'm separated from Wi-Fi, TV, the grind of the city, and the memories of Dan are replaced with maudlin cow moos, homecooked breakfasts and earthy, bucolic smells.

The course is taking place in the house once owned by poet laureate Ted Hughes, a native Yorkshireman who bequeathed the property to a literary charity. It's welly country up

THAT JOKE ISN'T FUNNY ANYMORE

here, no buses, no tubes, a mix of muddy browns and leafy greens; lunch is dinner, and dinner is tea, and everyone is chipper and unpretentious.

The house is austere, a mossy, weather-beaten building cast of pumis-grey stone. It's dark inside, with creaking oak floorboards, vast wooden beams overhead, low-ceilinged dining rooms, windows that rattle in the sharp northern wind.

There's ten of us here, all amateurs at various stages. Sharing meals on thick oak dining tables, talking story and character with my companions, the parallels between writing and mental health nursing seem stark. Both are to do with bringing order to chaos. Both can be funny, affirming, rewarding, but also painful, confusing, dogged with uncertainty.

By the end of the week I've scribbled out several thousand words. I've thought a lot. Met good people. Slept and laughed. Really, the last thing on my mind should've been a visit to the grave of Sylvia Plath, Ted Hughes' wife, whose suicide remains one of the saddest and most poignant in the annuls. But on learning that she was interred a short walk away, it seemed remiss to not go.

So it came to be that on the penultimate day before returning to London, I'm stood in St Thomas a Becket's churchyard beneath a grey slate of sky. As graves go, it's an unremarkable one. Sandy grey. Embossed black lettering. A simple Hindu epitaph. A beaker of writing pens left by an admirer sits against the stone, the receptacle filled with rainwater turned murky black from the ink. Gazing down, I'm unsure what I was expecting. Perhaps a flash of inspiration. Something to funnel into writing.

All that comes is the waste of it all. Plath died by placing her head in an oven while her children slept, a culmination of years of melancholia she fought against. Fifty years on, Dan had a similar battle with his demons. Both lost.

Now, as the rain drizzles down, it all seems clear to me.

I'm approaching forty. Dan's inquest is coming up. And I've hit an almighty brick wall.

'Mr Sweeney?' the coroner says.

I look at her, catapulted back to the present.

'Have you anything you'd like to add before we adjourn?'

'No,' I say.

'Does anyone from the deceased's family have anything to say?'

Simone, Dan's twin, peers up. Her green eyes are alit. For a second, I'm staring at him. She clears her throat. I'm sure she's about to berate me.

'Happy birthday,' she says.

After, in the sterile hallway leading out to St Pancras Gardens, she approaches.

'I found out from Dan,' she says, 'about your birthday. In case you're wondering how I knew it was today.'

'He told you?'

'He had it written down in his diary. The big four-oh, and your name. I guess he planned to send you a card. If he'd still been here, that is.'

I have no idea what to say.

'That coroner gave you a hard time, but there was nothing you could've done. I know that.'

Nod.

'He'd have found all this funny. You having to come here when you should be eating birthday cake. Try to remember the good times.'

'He said something similar.'

'There you go.'

As the hallway empties, she goes on to tell me things about Dan that should remain unsaid. At the end, I leave her my phone number – probably a bad idea – and offer to meet if she'd like to. She says that'd be nice.

But she doesn't call. And I'm glad.

This is just a phase, I tell myself – keep calm and carry on. But attempts at self-reassurance fall limp. I'm ready to chuck in the towel with mental health nursing.

Not just because of Dan. In the past year I've become jaded. Phrases like therapeutic intervention, behavioural activation, motivational interviewing – they sound good on paper but I'm starting to wonder if psychiatry is pseudoscience, namby-pamby, rubbish.

An example: a few months prior, I'd witnessed an on-call middle-grade psychiatrist get badgered by an anxious nurse to assess a patient admitted to an orthopaedic ward. On top of a leg fracture, this patient was apparently in a state of psychosis. Said psychiatrist dutifully ventured up.

Half an hour later he returned, confirming that the patient was indeed floridly psychotic, trying to mask symptoms, lacking insight, and posed a grave risk to herself.

'Himself?' the nurse said. 'The patient I asked you to see is a man.'

It transpired the psychiatrist had examined the patient

on Bay 12, not Bay 11: the woman he'd been convinced was unwell, masking symptoms, a grave danger, was fine and dandy.

This harks back to the renown Rosenhan Experiment from the early 1970s that dismantled the validity of psychiatry in a swoop. A group of mentally 'well' individuals entered a series of facilities across the States, all claiming to hear in their heads a cluster of random words like 'thud'. These claims led to enforced admissions, diagnoses of psychosis – and great difficulty getting discharged when the individuals revealed they'd been faking. The study showed how subjective and inaccurate mental health diagnostic criteria can be. It was funny and shocking and fed into the narrative that psychiatry was a sham.

Right now, it seems like a sham to me. And a dangerous sham for those with careers in it. Recent data from NHS England shows more than 1.5 million nurse days were lost in 2022 due to anxiety, stress, depression and other psychiatric illnesses – on average, one in five of every sickness days was due to mental ill health. A similar study by the Royal College of Nursing shows a spike in suicidal thoughts and stress-related resignations among mental health professionals, significantly higher than national averages. Google 'mental health problems in mental health professionals' and you'll be faced with a grim and lengthy read.

I've seen nurses like Dan who've had to leave because the job gets too much. Burnout, compassion fatigue, vicarious traumas – like he said, the stories we hear seep into us and metastasize, and become a threat to our own sanity. How many tales of incest, abuse, rape, suicide attempts and self-harm is it possible to hear? Many times I've come home feeling dirty, used up.

It's patently obvious. Writers get writers' block. Marathon runners hit the runners' wall. And mental health nurses get depressed and top themselves.

In the acclaimed *Save the Cat* storytelling rulebook, this would be the 'Dark Night of the Soul' beat of my career. With Radiohead playing in the background, there'd be a protracted scene of me on the top deck of a bus, looking mournfully from the window, brooding and mulling, grappling with whether to remain a mental health nurse.

I have options – a friend from the gym works in finance and offers to share my resume with his colleagues; I've got a mate who's branched out into software programming, another who's become an estate agent. Could I see myself doing something like them?

They're intriguing ideas. But I don't take them up. And I'm glad for it. If I'd quit, I wouldn't have penned this book. Instead, something Dan said pings like an unread text.

Write about the job.

Charles Bukowski said that writing is the best psychiatrist there is. It was time to find out.

An intersection of themes presents itself. How about a detective novel told through a mental health lens? What Raymond Chandler might've written had he done my peculiar job in twenty-first century London. And what if my protagonist had his life torn up by suicide? His quest isn't to solve a crime, but to make some sense of his own unbearable loss.

It takes the best part of a year to get the manuscript into decent shape. Writing every day before work. Editing at lunchtime. Refining late into the night until fatigue claims me. By the end, I have an 80,000-word draft and know I have something half-decent. And to my surprise, while writing, the pull to leave mental health nursing has dissipated.

It's corny – writing saved me! But the truth is, through the process I was able to reframe some of the madness, gain distance and give a salute to Dan along the way. Looking back, I'm pretty sure writing has made me a better nurse. And I'm certain nursing has made me a better writer.

Renewed, with a book to pitch, Spencer walking, talking, fast outgrowing our tiny flat, Clare and I begin making plans for our big move to the northwest. Life, it seems, is back on course.

As if.

Around this time, news of a strange bug from China hits the news. Then, while I'm having tentative talks with a literary agent, people start to lose their sense of taste and develop nasty, persistent coughs.

Suffer the Children

'DAMMIT,' I SAY, as the third facemask of the day snaps over my ear.

Daisy, fifteen, immersed in her smartphone, doesn't seem to notice.

We're in her bedroom, situated in a mid-terraced house in a part of central Lancashire I'd never heard of until a few weeks back. Although it's afternoon, Daisy's wearing a dressing gown and pyjamas, both emblazoned with Elsa from *Frozen*. A wiry teenager, she's crossed-legged on her bed. The dressing gown hood is up. Wool socks are pulled tight over her feet. She cradles her smartphone with the affection I used to show my teddy bear.

'What was I talking about?' I say, fishing a fresh mask from my pocket.

'Me,' Daisy says, her voice light and husky from underuse. 'How you're going to help.'

'Right,' I say.

In truth, I haven't a clue what to do with this reclusive,

erudite girl who hasn't left her bedroom in over a year. She's neurodivergent, with high-functioning autism, and struggles with anxiety, depression and suicidal ideas. Primary school was manageable, but secondary school, where the angst, conflict and comparisons kicked in, had a scolding effect. Then Covid landed. Schools closed. Like thousands of adolescents across the UK, Daisy took to her room. And she hasn't come out since.

'What your parents want,' I say, 'is for you to gain confidence. To come out a bit and socialise.'

'I *do* socialise,' she says, and holds up the smartphone. 'My friends are on this.'

I'd walked into that one. Dale, her dad, gave her the iPhone a couple of years back, late compared to some of her peers, who'd had phones since primary school. For Dale, the phone was a way to keep in touch and give her greater independence. A help.

Her slight finger scrolls on the screen. The colours flash luridly off her eyes like lit-up slot machines.

'What are you looking at?' I say.

'Just an app,' she answers.

'Want to tell me about it?'

'Nah.'

'Why not?'

'You wouldn't get it.'

'How do you know?'

'You're out of touch.'

'I'm not,' I say with a laugh.

Daisy doesn't answer.

Am I out of touch?

Her bedroom is much like any other teenage girl's – Taylor Swift and Yungblud posters, a Nintendo Switch on a dresser, fake eyelashes, bronzer, schoolbooks and exercise pads strewn about. But there is a sadness here too, evident in the drawn curtains, the dimmed lights, the wardrobe mirror that's been covered with a towel to avoid catching a reflection.

So far, I've suggested we go for a walk round the block, take the dog out, go to the shop and aim to visit her school, where the kids are beginning to return; I've told her about graded exposure, small steps towards meeting goals, the stuff I've done with adults, hoping it might chime. Throughout, she's stayed inert, beholden to the screen.

I check my watch. I've been here twenty minutes and have got nowhere. 'I'll drop by in a fortnight then,' I say.

It's as if I don't exist.

Downstairs, I describe to Dale, a joiner by trade, the conversation I've just had with his daughter. It doesn't take long.

'She's always been a quiet one,' he says, his northern accent pronounced, the vowels drawn out. 'She keeps herself to herself. But this is a whole new level. Not going out. Not talking to anyone. We're worried she's going to do something. Right, love?' He looks at Lianne, his wife, sitting at the dining room table, nursing a brew.

'Do you think you can help her?' she says.

'Well,' I say, 'I'll keep trying.'

'It's taken us a year to get CAMHS to send you. She's not left the room that whole time. Please do all you can. We're relying on you.'

I tell them I'll do my best, and leave the house, where my recently bought Vauxhall Corsa is parked outside.

It's raining. When I hit the ignition, the satnav on my phone is having trouble connecting. I look up at the gunmetal sky of the northwest and begin driving, hoping I'll recognise where I am.

But I don't; and as I meander around cobbled streets with names I've never heard of, the rain blasts, lashing and beating, and it occurs to me that I *am* out of touch, with my new job, my new area, my life—

A jolt as my car mounts a chevron. I pull the wheel left, and almost clip a Land Rover's wing mirror. With my heart in my throat, I drive on, trying to stay calm, focus on what's on the road, not how strange life seems.

Then I see the blue lights behind me. The police. I pull up to the kerb, dejected.

A minute later, I'm standing beside my car, cold and wet, breathing into a breathalyser before a fresh-faced young constable. When my alcohol reading comes back negative, he tells me to 'Stay safe', and that I'm free to go.

But I don't go. As the police pull away I stay in the pelting rain, seeing my life before me. It's Covid. I'm working with a client group I know nothing about, in a town, a county, a region that's alien to me.

Noticing I haven't moved, the constable turns his car around and pulls up beside me. I stare down, shiver. He lowers the window, says, 'Are you lost, Sir?'

I tell him I do believe I am.

✻

SUFFER THE CHILDREN

Many years before, a nurse I knew said that her career in children's mental health services was the best form of birth control – if you do it, you won't ever want kids of your own. I laughed at the time, but the remark stuck in my head. Now, in my adopted home in the northwest, I find myself poised to test out its accuracy.

Like many Londoners, I considered anything past the Watford Junction as 'the North', and it all looked much of a muchness. Grey skies. Muddy roads. Funny accents. Rain. Then I married a Northerner and got an education. It's a stereotype, but Northerners are a friendlier bunch. Strangers say hello to each other on the streets. Do that in London, they'll think you're a mugger. There isn't the rat race so much up here, that chase for status and property.

After Spencer came, the advantages of a move screamed out. Cheaper living. Grandparents close by. Less pollution, knife crime, phone snatchers, bike thieves, cramped accommodation and skyrocketing living costs.

Covid was the impetus. During those lockdown days, life became a dystopia. Supermarket shelves ransacked, a national shortage of toilet paper, people panic-buying, preparing for a pandemic winter. Camden High Street, Archway Road, Piccadilly Circus became desolate, populated only by the homeless, dispossessed, the marginalised, the lost. Strange new laws appeared, who you could and couldn't see, how much time you were allowed out, how far you could and could not go from your home. Weird elbow touches replaced handshakes, terms like 'super-spreader' and 'stay safe' did the rounds, and every night on TV came the death stats. Who next?

Working in mental health through the pandemic was particularly odd. Several colleagues caught the bug and went off. Others who had pre-existing conditions were told to shield. A few quit, or refused to come in. One nurse I knew got sick and died.

The rest of us were considered essential workers. But whereas our colleagues working in general health were being battered by respiratory patients flooding A&E, in community mental health there was a feeling of uncertainty, malaise, not quite knowing what to do. Guidelines stipulated we should avoid face-to-face contact, swapping in-person appointments with phone or video calls, keeping tabs on patients through 'telepsychiatry'.

I struggled with this. Working as a mental health nurse is about human connections, not sterile digital interfaces. Some patients were tech-savvy but many weren't, not having smartphones, not being able to afford them or not knowing how they worked. For some, the loneliness and enforced isolation fed into anxiety and depression, and they sank; for others, the conspiracy theories and surveillance reports hitting the news were like petrol to the sparks of paranoia.

We did our best, making phone and video calls to support them through this Groundhog Day, wondering when it would end. For those whose mental health was in decline, we visited, clad in masks, aprons, and gloves worn like coats of armour. When not contacting patients, the job became a planning one, arranging food parcels and medication deliveries to those who couldn't venture out; making daily welfare calls to a long list of patients, checking they were OK. It was heartwarming to witness the volume of grassroots support that emerged, charities and everyday folk banding together to help. On the flipside, the pandemic put a spotlight on the shoddy resources and unequipped crisis plans engrained in the NHS, with its dearth of PPE, laptops and testing equipment for us to use.

We tried to put a cheery spin on things, muddling together as a team to maintain a wartime spirit, buoyed by the public support. Thursday evenings, people came out and clapped for us NHS heroes; Pret A Manger put up free coffees and croissants for those carrying a hospital ID. Yet none of it could dislodge that pinch of existential doom that coloured everything. Was this really the 'new normal'?

Catastrophes, I told myself, are why I joined the health service – to do my bit to help others. When word circulated that us nurses would be redeployed to general hospitals, freeing shortfalls due to sicknesses, allowing specialists to be sent to the new Nightingale units, I was ready for it. But this, like so much during the period, never materialised. Instead, the miasma of doubt cloyed in the air.

London didn't seem like London anymore. It was during the second lockdown that Clare and I made the decision to stick a compass in a map of the northwest, do a few online viewings with estate agents, find a place we liked near a decent primary school, and go for it.

Now it's a fortnight since that big move. We have ourselves a charming semi-detached home with a drive out front, a back garden needing work, and we've enrolled Spencer into a local nursery. Home is a provincial seaside town synonymous with its coastal fairs, the home of Les Dawson, Bobby Ball, golf courses, care homes and a slow, steady lifestyle. Locals are smiley and friendly. The *Mail* is the paper of choice.

Everyone has a dog. And everyone scoops up after said dog. Wood Green High Street this is not.

Lying in bed that first night, I was struck by the sound coming from outside. At first, I couldn't tell what it was. Then it clicked. Nothing. I couldn't hear a peep.

I'd applied for a few jobs in the preceding weeks, keeping options open, not being picky. The Child and Adolescent Mental Health Services (CAMHS) position I accepted was the most intriguing. My colleague's remark all those years ago came back. Was working with young people really that bad? Course not. After the year we'd just had, supporting angsty northern teenagers should be a doddle.

Right?

'My three-year-old son's a whizz with my smartphone.'

Daisy, for the first time, looks up from her screen.

'He's three. He likes dinosaur sites and Lego sites and watching YouTube shorts of kids his age unwrapping toys and playing with them before opening more toys and chucking them around the place.'

'I know that stream,' Daisy says, in the same light voice as before. With the stealth of a flautist, she taps onto her screen, holds it up, and shows me the latest upload.

'Yup,' I say, 'that's the one.'

For a minute, the vacuous video plays out: two boys tearing apart boxes of toys in front of their gormless, grinning mum. It's pure ephemera. When I wince, Daisy giggles. Although her face is starved of sunlight and vitamin D, she's striking – elfish, androgenous, with sloping eyes, a sharp nose and thin pink lips.

'What do you like looking at on your phone?' I ask when it's finished.

She skims through her apps. There are the usual suspects – Insta, TikTok, YouTube, Snapchat, Facebook – but there's ones I haven't heard of, with strange, one-word names that allow for anonymous messaging and multiuser chat. When I enquire what Daisy uses them for, there's a recurring theme: communication.

'It's how I keep in touch with the world,' she says.

'What about going out?'

'I don't need to go out.'

Behind my mask, my face is galvanised with shock.

'Mind if I sit?' I ask.

Daisy gestures towards a chair covered in clothes. Carefully, I remove them, place them on the carpet, conscious of my size, my gender, the age gap, and how odd I look hidden in latex gloves, a crinkly apron and the mask.

'Maybe you should be looking at other things,' I say, 'apart from your phone.'

'Chloe said you'd say that.'

'Chloe?'

'My friend.'

'How long have you known her?'

'Two weeks.'

'You've met her? In person?'

Daisy shrugs.

'Where does she live?'

'New York.'

'How old is she?'

'Same as me.'

'You're sure she is who she says she is?'

'We're soul sisters. She's had problems. Like me. With bullying. She was thinking about suicide too.'

Immediately, my safeguarding antenna pings. I've read about chatrooms aimed at teens, unregulated, open grounds for undesirables to lure and groom. Daisy's proficiency with technology is matched by her naivety. What is this stuff doing to her sponge of a mind?

'Chloe's helped me,' she says.

'How has Chloe helped?'

'She's my friend.'

'Friends meet up in real life.'

'You don't know what it's like being my age.'

I scoff, remembering David Bowie's lyrics from his song 'Changes' about kids being 'immune to your consultations'. I recite the lines to Daisy.

'It's by Bowie.'

'Who's Bowie?'

Before I can answer, a message pings up on her phone, harpooning her away: *Who's Bowie?*

I'd never considered myself old.

Till now.

'Have you talked about taking her phone away?' I ask Dale. 'She thinks she's using it to make friends, but it's clearly harming her.'

We're in the kitchen, like before. Dale looks at Lianne, seated at the table. A cautious look passes between them, as if I've mentioned a recently departed friend.

'What?' I say.

'We've tried taking the phone,' Dale says.

'But Daisy,' Lianne adds, 'she gets so crabby, so we let her have it.'

'It's all she's got,' Dale adds, apologetically.

'And that's what's making her lonely and isolated and the way she is.'

I'm starting to get crabby too. These parents are enabling their daughter to remain stuck.

Dale shrugs, a what-can-you-do? expression. Lianne stares at her mug of tea.

I leave, pulling off my PPE with as much bluster as the act permits.

CAMHS work, I discover, involves lots of people. Along with psychiatrists, psychologists, nurses, social workers, psychotherapists, family therapists and occupational therapists on my team, there are the parents, siblings, teachers, social services, neighbours, priests, police – all with opinions, often wildly different, about what needs to happen to help the child in question with their mental health.

Many referrals fail to meet the stringent criteria needed to access help. Instead, the youngster gets signposted to social services, the voluntary sector, back to the GP, or rejected full stop. Those few that are allowed in will generally go to the bottom of one of several hefty waiting lists where they sit, like Daisy's referral did, for upwards of a year to be seen.

There are kids with anxiety, depression, self-harm, suicidal ideation – many of the disorders I'm familiar with from the adult sector already taking root in burgeoning teenagers. ADHD is a regular cause for enquiry too, with many parents concerned that their unruly, distractable child has a neurodivergence.

Then there's the scourge of social media to contend with.

Times are different to when I was a kid. Sure, we got angsty about relationships, school, bodies, love lives. But this proliferation of smartphones, high-speed internet and social media apps is brand new, and seems to have rewired children's brains. Rather than being a tool for education and growth, many blame the ubiquity as being the foremost reason for today's disconnection, disillusion and dysphoria.

There are bundles of evidence to support this. A recent report by the University of North Carolina found that teens who habitually checked social media experienced quantifiable changes in the neurotransmission in the frontal cortexes. Said changes were linked to emotional regulation, management of frustration, social interaction and how peer feedback is received. In other words, the more time adolescents – especially vulnerable ones – spend online, the higher the levels of eating disorders, depression, anxiety, suicidality and general misery prevail.

In the UK this has led to a growing pressure to police social media for the sake of our kids. As I write, a leading school academy trust is set to put a complete ban on mobile phone use among students during the school day. Likewise, in February 2024, Esther Ghey attended Parliament to call for a smartphone ban for under-sixteens and insisted the Online Safety Act fails to protect teenagers. Ghey, mother of Brianna, who was murdered by two teenagers – one of whom was a prolific viewer of torture sites on the dark web – criticised existing safeguards for failing to prevent real-life tragedies.

But those who support reform are up against a tsunami of opposition. The tech firms have algorithms that are money-making mutants. Meta, the giant behind Facebook, insists it has removed much of the content related to suicide, self-harm and eating disorders. But it was too late for Molly Russell, a fourteen-year-old who took her life after viewing reams of online pages about suicide. During the inquest, the coroner drew irrefutable links between her death and this unhealthy interest the internet allowed her to explore. Is Daisy at risk of going down the same route?

Some of my new CAMHS colleagues suggest I maintain a softly-softly approach with her, visiting regularly, slowly trying to build rapport. Some think I should act assertively, insisting her parents implement boundaries and wrench her from her bedroom. Everyone agrees that Daisy's absorption in her phone is the main obstacle.

That afternoon, back at the team's office, a grey, prosaic health centre on a main road in Blackpool, I dip my toe into a few of the apps Daisy showed me. Before long I'm shocked at the profanity, the pornography, the promotion of cruelty and illness that populate them all. The chatrooms are particularly bitchy – comments about acne, cellulite, bad teeth, weight comparisons, self-harming and suicide are tossed out as freely as a croupier dealing cards.

Hoping for reassurance that this isn't standard fare, I speak to Daisy's class teacher, a newly qualified young man, clearly committed to his vocation:

'This pandemic – it's got a lot to answer for. Suddenly,

schools close, kids get sent home, and are encouraged to rely on technology and the internet to communicate.'

'Do you think that's what caused Daisy's problems?' I ask.

'There were issues before Covid,' he says. 'But it's got worse now. She's in a slump, not submitting course work, not engaging at all. She won't get any GCSEs at this rate. It's sad. She's a dead bright girl.'

'Any advice?'

'Get her off that phone.'

I video-call Daisy's social worker, a no-nonsense woman who has a smoker's cough and Su Pollard specs. Her feedback is much the same:

'Yeah, she's a good kid, but she's stuck in a rut now. And her parents, God love them, they've not been firm. Let Daisy walk over them.'

'Any advice?'

'Try to get her out. And off that bloody phone.'

I decide to follow the advice, call Dale and Lianne and tell them that for Daisy to improve and get over her agoraphobia they need to be tough: she needs to be prised away from the smartphone. It's the only way.

'But she'll hate us,' Dale says.

'Maybe for a bit,' I say. 'Hopefully in the future, she'll realise why you did it.'

There's a pause.

'You think it'll work?'

'Yes,' I say.

Although, truth be told, I already have a bad feeling.

*

A week later, that feeling grows teeth.

It's an afternoon in early spring. I'm working from home, having just picked Spencer up from his nursery, where the staff still wear face masks at half-mast, like a token.

It's been a dull day – screening referrals, phoning GPs, calling parents, all from the confines of my lounge, as we're still discouraged from face-to-face meetings and instead work from home. I'm wearing the standard Covid WFH uniform. On my top half, an ironed shirt; while my bottom half, out of sight for video calls, is barely clad in three-stripe Adidas shorts. When my phone starts ringing, I prise it away from Spencer, who has already figured out the eight-digit pin-code and how to access games. The caller is Dale, Daisy's dad.

'She's in hospital,' he says. The line is bad, a lot of background noise. Dale, in an A&E department, shouts down the receiver about what took place.

That morning, he found Daisy collapsed on the carpet of her bedroom, foaming at the mouth. Empty boxes of paracetamol were scattered around her. Her pulse was weak.

'How is she?' I say.

'They say she'll pull through,' Dale says.

There is a pause. Spencer stares up at me keenly, knowing something is amiss.

'What happened?' I say, although I already know the answer.

'We did like you said,' Dale says. 'We took away her phone.'

The overdose wasn't enough to kill Daisy, and the Parvolex and IV fluids they pump through clear the toxic effects.

While she's hooked up to the machines, they also shove in vitamins, iron and decent nutrition, none of which she'd have got otherwise.

But once medically cleared, there is concern that she might do something similar. Dale has found reams of websites on her phone – all pro-suicide – giving advice and instructions to the novice about the ways and arrangements needed to get the job done.

After a back and forth, it's agreed that Daisy should be admitted to the local CAMHS inpatient unit for a period of assessment and formulation. An ambulance drives her and her parents there later that day.

Adolescent mental health units share similarities with their adult equivalents – they're secure, meaning doors are locked, and they tend to have a greyness about their facade that screams 'institution'. Some patients will be kept there voluntarily, whereas others will be detained; the staff will come from a range of backgrounds, from psychiatrists and medical doctors to psychologists, occupational therapists, dieticians and nurses; they are noisy, scary, inspiring, depressing and provocative places. But the buoyancy of youth adds an extra pinch of spice.

Because patients are of school age, there must be the provision of OFSTED-inspected education, delivered either by visiting teachers or through online portals. Moreso than with adult wards, adolescent units will have an emphasis on talking therapies, ideally involving the parents, and delivered in a systemic manner, looking at the family unit and how each member plays a role in the problem, and the solution.

In my experience, inpatient CAMHS nurses are some of

the coolest, most opinionated and at times cantankerous on our workforce. With the proliferation of combat boots, tats, piercings and pronouns, you'd be forgiven for thinking you'd walked into a hipster nightclub, not a mental health ward. When I visit CAMHS units, I'm regularly impressed by these nurses' innate ability to communicate with their patients, find commonality, show patience, talk their language. It's a job I couldn't do.

When I next see Daisy, it's a couple of days into the admission and she's in the communal lounge of the unit. Magnolia walls, lilac carpets and embraided pillows add some colour to the fire-retardant sofas and armchairs. LGBTQ+ support groups, Childline, sexual health drop-ins, teenage advocacy, all postered around the walls next to magazine cut-outs of popstars. I've heard of a few – Dua Lipa, Wet Leg, Billie Eilish. The rest are just names.

There are four other teenagers in this lounge, each splayed out on the furniture, dressed in loose sports clothes, looking inward and serious. Two nurses lean against the walls – one male, one I can't be sure – recognisable for their NHS lanyards and face masks.

Daisy's Elsa dressing gown dwarves her. She is on a sofa, staring ahead. Without her phone, her hands are twined together, squeezing, scratching, plucking, as if the fingers are unsure what to do with themselves.

'Hiya,' I say, sitting on a fire-retardant footrest opposite. 'You're looking well.'

She nods, but she doesn't look at me. 'They've taken my phone,' she says. 'Mum and Dad.'

'I heard.'

'Did you tell them to do that?'

'I suggested you were spending too much time on it.'

A girl on the sofa to the left sniggers.

'Want to talk about what happened?' I say.

'I took some pills.'

'Why did you take them?'

'Because Mum and Dad took my phone.'

'Why did they take your phone?'

'Because I was spending too much time on it. Then they found the sites I was looking at. Ones about taking pills.'

'Exactly,' I say, spotting an inlet. 'Don't you see that this might be a good thing?'

The other girl sniggers again. 'Told you he'd say that,' she says.

I ignore her. 'Hopefully, you won't be here long.'

Daisy shrugs.

'They aren't real friends you've made online, you must realise that.'

She nods. 'Yeah. Not real friends. Not like Steph.'

'Steph?'

The girl to the left stands and comes to sit beside Daisy. I take her in. She's short, stocky, built like an XL Bully; I'd put her about seventeen, but she's already weathered, with bad teeth, a buzz cut, her expression sharpened with an 'and what?' stare. Self-harm scars on her arms look deep and permanent. Bad news is written all over her.

'Hello, Steph,' I say.

She smiles, a yellow, hateful smile, and then she whispers something to Daisy. The remark is about me, I can tell; and from Daisy's grin, it isn't flattering.

'I'm going to my room now,' she says. 'Steph, come on.'

The two girls stand, begin walking. I look at the nurses, hoping they will intervene. But how can they? They aren't doing anything wrong.

'Shall I come back and see you next week?' I call.

'No,' Daisy says, and is gone.

Steph, I learn, is a regular at the hospital. She had her first admission aged thirteen after she overdosed on cocaine her inebriated stepdad left out. Since then, there have been over a dozen more.

Now seventeen, she's on a full care order with the local authority and has been from placement to placement up and down the country. The longest lasted three months, ending when she started a fire in her bedroom after being asked to turn her music down. Since then, fifteen young person's accommodation providers have refused to house her – arsonists tend to get a bad rep.

Prior to this admission, she was living in an Airbnb with two support workers in situ 24/7. Despite the intensive support, neither seemed able to keep her from acquiring razors and self-harming badly enough to wind up in A&E again, and then getting sent to the same unit as Daisy.

Steph, now on the cusp of adulthood, is already a mental health veteran. She prefers hospital to living out in the community, knows the system, understands how to get admitted, what to say and do. Patients like her get a bad press, for they generate anxiety and drain resources. But if you look at her history, the chaos she's borne from, it's easy to see why she's the way she is.

Normally, I'd sympathise, see her as a victim, a child let down. But other things are taking precedence. Worryingly, Steph appears to have formed a deep impression on Daisy.

In the fortnight that follows, Daisy leans into Steph, and closes the door on me. When I visit again, she stays in her room. When I call, she won't speak to me. Instead, I learn from nursing staff that Steph is her confidante, soulmate, BFF and mentor. Sure enough, Daisy soon learns to conceal her prescribed antidepressants in her gums, self-harm with sharpened crayons and moulded cutlery, fashion bed sheets and pillowcases into ligatures; she becomes mouthy with staff, screaming, hurling abuse, making threats of the kind Steph is renowned for.

It's clear the admission is creating more problems than it's fixing, and discharge is on the cards – but that might not be easy. Before long, the word is out that she and Steph have made a suicide pact.

'I thought Daisy's meant to get better in hospital,' Dale says to me over the phone when I tell him this.

'I know,' I say. 'I mean, hopefully she still will get better. This is a little . . . unexpected.'

In truth, it isn't so uncommon – contagion is a recognised social phenomenon. In clinical settings, it defines the passing of diseases from one to another, and with organic illness like coughs and colds, the transmission is through germs and bacteria. In mental health, it's a little more nuanced, shared through emulation, copycat-ing, encouragement, coercion, and a weird kind of psychic osmosis.

I'm left feeling useless. When I applied to work with children and adolescents, my aim was to support young people, intervene sooner, and help them avoid developing problems as adults. Never would I have envisioned the system I'm part of could make them worse.

The next three months are a strange time. While Covid restrictions gradually lift, and social anxiety begins to dampen, my attempts to support Daisy enter a new phase.

A decision is made by senior NHS managers that the two girls – Daisy and Steph – need separating. Steph has a residential placement lined up in the Midlands that the council have agreed to fork out for. Daisy can return to her family. A hundred miles separating the two girls, the geographical distance will eliminate their suicide pact. What could go wrong?

On a warm Monday in May, Steph boards a taxi taking her to the placement in Solihull. A few hours later, Daisy's parents pick her up. Around teatime, I check in with them.

'She's OK,' Dale says hesitantly, adding, 'but she's back in her room, and back on her phone.'

'You gave Daisy her phone?' I can't hide the dismay in my voice.

'Well, yes,' he says. 'I mean, she wanted it. Maybe she'll have learned something from all this?'

By Tuesday, Daisy's gone. Her parents report her missing. They are, understandably, in bits. I don my professional hat, try telling them the police are looking for her, they know what they're doing, but we all think the worst. Right now, Daisy is hanging somewhere.

No body emerges.

Instead, there are extensive searches, helicopters, dogs, local then national alerts, all the whistles and bells. A little after midnight, a girl wearing a distinctive *Frozen* dressing gown is spotted on a platform in Birmingham New Street Station, pale, shivery, trying to find somewhere to charge her phone. When police compare her to a photofit, they know it's Daisy. Turns out she was trying to figure out which connecting train will take her to Solihull.

'Your parents were worried sick,' I say the following morning after the police have dropped her home. She's in her bedroom, cross-legged on the mattress once more. Her phone has been taken away. She looks bereft. 'What were you trying to do?'

'I was going to see Steph.'

'Did you find her?'

'She stood me up.'

'There you go. Steph's not your friend.'

'Can you get my phone back?'

'No.' With facemasks non-mandatory, Daisy can see my exasperation.

'You're mean,' she says. Her eyes well up.

I'm aware of a headache clawing. 'Are you going to run off again?' I ask, putting some softness into my voice.

'No.'

'Promise?'

'Promise.'

But she does.

Over the next few weeks, a pattern emerges. For a day or two, things are calm. Then she goes missing, gets reported to the police, and is eventually found at random locations up and down the country. At first, the police are sympathetic, bringing her home, remonstrating with Dale and Lianne. Before long, though, Daisy gains a reputation as a time-waster and gets treated with disregard. Rather than take her home, police deposit her in paediatric emergency departments where staff must call Security to keep her.

There are multiple assessments and disagreements about what should happen. The CAMHS inpatient unit point-blank refuses to readmit her, saying Daisy's problems are social and further admission could be counterproductive. The consensus is that community CAMHS – specifically me – should be doing more.

And I'd like to do more. But despite my adherence to all the Covid rules, my acceptance of the jabs and PPE, I find myself developing a chesty cough . . .

About the time I'm testing positive for the bug, Daisy is in a general hospital, held down by Security to stop her leaving; some unscrupulous patient videos her writhing around and it ends up on YouTube like the scene from *The Exorcist* of the demon girl. Wallowing in my sick bed, it feels as if this is somehow my fault.

Strategy meetings follow. In vast MS Teams meetings, senior people with letters after their names bluster and point at me: 'You're from CAMHS?'

'Yes,' I croak.

'What are you doing about this?'

I'm in the dark. Whatever connection I had with Daisy seems to have disintegrated. I'm as clueless as anyone, completely out of touch.

'It was better when she was in her bedroom,' Dale says to

me over the phone a week later, as I emerge from isolation. 'At least we could keep tabs on her.'

'Yes,' I say. My voice has returned but my lungs feel like they're full of wet cement.

'I wish we'd never asked for help. It's made her worse.'

He's right.

If the CAMHS team I'm a part of were in good condition, I'd perhaps be more spirited. But the fact is the service is collapsing too – walkouts, sicknesses, stress, managers coming one minute, going the next; I've had scant supervision, no reassurance, and even less guidance since I started. When the third manager walks, a senior reaches out and suggests I might go for the post. Politely, I reply that I cannot think of anything worse.

It's a dark time. Clare and I consider moving back to London.

But we don't. Up here, we have a nice house, family near, and our son is settled. Like it or not, this is home for the foreseeable.

One small nugget of positivity from this time is that an idea for my second novel emerges. Struck by the disturbing power imbued in a smartphone, this idea then moulds into a plot about real-life barbarity getting captured and circulated online for sadistic glee. Although dark, writing the story helps create some sense in this strange chapter in my career.

But mostly, it's grim. Rachel Reeves MP recently stated that it's tougher for kids today than it used to be. I agree. There are things they experience, influences they're exposed to through the digital age, that even a thick-skinned mental health professional like me is shocked at.

The good news is that Daisy and Steph don't fulfil the suicide pact. Instead, Steph starts another fire in her new placement, this one growing into a pyre, which leads to her getting arrested and being remanded at a young offender institution, pending a court date, taking her out of the picture. Before long, Daisy returns to her room. With her smartphone. And regresses like before.

The final time I see her, I'm telling her that I'm quitting my job. She's cross-legged on her bed like the first time we met, swamped in a new *Frozen* dressing gown, her phone in her hands. I'm expecting her to blank me. Instead, she stops scrolling and her eyes become wet.

'Will you still visit?' There's surprise in her voice.

'Why?' I say.

She shrugs.

'You'll get a new care coordinator,' I say. 'Someone else will take my place.'

She nods slowly.

'Well,' I say, 'take care.'

'Hold on.'

Her mouth opens. I'm willing her to offer something real.

'Can I add you to my Insta?' she says.

Two things happen after that. I don't see Daisy again. And I vow never to work in CAMHS again either.

That was a few years ago. Now I hear it on good authority that Daisy has shown improvements. She's dropped the Elsa dressing gown, dyed her hair and has ventured out with her parents, applying to go to college to study animal care. Why it happened this way is a mystery. Maybe she had a moment of clarity and saw the harm she was inflicting. Maybe the support she was given had a delayed impact. Or maybe she just changed, growing and maturing the way young people are supposed to.

That evening, sitting in the lounge with Spencer on my lap, I draft a resignation letter explaining that I've reached the conclusion that CAMHS work isn't for me. As a caveat, I'm tempted to include the famous line from Larkin's lauded poem, 'This Be The Verse', about what your mum and dad do, but don't mean to. I can't recall all the verses. Instinctively, I reach for my iPhone. As the screen lights up, Spencer's eyes are snared, and he snatches the phone away.

'Hey,' I say.

Oblivious, he begins swiping and scrolling, his three-year-old's tiny fingers moving with disconcerting ease. Part of me is marvelled at his wizardry at such a young age. But another part of me is grieving the loss of innocence these strange rectangular objects represent.

I scrap the poem quote, hit send on my resignation, and then watch Spencer, screen to face, his eyes wide and blinking like the shutters of a camera.

Some Girls are Bigger than Others

IT'S A CLOSE, muggy day in mid-July, and Rachel, twenty-two, is busy explaining to two psychiatrists and me the reasons why she's lost a further 300 grams of weight since being admitted to a general hospital: 'It's because they put too much salt in the food here,' she says, fastidiously. 'It's revolting. Honestly, I like eating. I do. But I can't bear what they serve. Yuck! That's why I've lost a bit more.'

As Rachel speaks, the pear-drops scent on her breath sweetens the air, a surefire sign that her body has entered ketosis and is starving. She's wearing an oversized Adidas tracksuit and All Stars. Her body looks pre-pubescent, but her face, bone pale, is old before its time. It gives her a stark incongruity, as if she's an elderly child.

Rachel collapsed three days ago. She should've been resting in bed due to her low blood pressure and anaemia. Instead, she'd been jogging and star-jumping on the spot.

I say, 'The notes suggest you're trying to avoid eating.

You've been observed drinking litres of water before being weighed, exercising and avoiding food. Staff are concerned.'

I'm being diplomatic. The handover we received from the charge nurse evidences that since Rachel came in she's been going to great lengths to dispose of, hide, give away or destroy the meals and meal replacements that have been brought to her. Nurses have found scrunched-up food hidden in the bed mattress, the curtains; they've seen her palming other patients with food, flushing food down the toilet, hiding food beneath her toenails, behind her ears, in her hair; they even suspect her of concealing food internally.

Presently, Rachel is bradycardic (low heart rate), anaemic (low iron levels) and has erratic blood pressure causing the fainting. She hasn't menstruated in two years, hasn't opened her bowels in a week, and is showing early signs of liver and kidney illness. The prognosis is bleak, and she's surely dying. Yet she thinks she's doing fine.

'I *am* fine,' she says, leaning in. 'All I want is to go home, back to Mum, and get on with my life.'

'Do you think you're overweight?' one of the psychiatrists behind me asks.

Rachel laughs, a confident, churlish sound. 'When I was younger, I did. Don't most girls? But I soon got over that.'

'Do you think you're a little too thin now?'

She laughs again. 'Well, a bit. But I'm sorting that out. Working with my dietician. Taking supplements.'

'What do you think would happen if you left the hospital?' I say.

'Nothing,' she snaps, as if I've asked a silly question. 'I'd go back to how I was. Me and Mum.'

I nod.

'So can I go now?'

Rachel's attempts to normalise her illness are convincing. In my experience, the anorexic mind can seduce and mislead better than the top MI5 agents. But the evidence before us is irrefutable, as clear as the fluorescent strip light buzzing above us in Rachel's hospital room. She's ill. Her mental disorder is distorting her mind and destroying her body.

In the hallway, the two psychiatrists and I have a discussion. We're all on the same page: Rachel needs to be kept here on the general ward and force-fed to save her life. This might sound severe – hell, it is severe, involving a nasal-gastric tube being inserted that can pump in liquidised meal replacements. In a different context, intrusive acts like these would be considered assault, bodily harm, barbaric. But in this context, under the umbrella of mental health legislation, it is defined as treatment. And right now, this treatment is the only way of being sure that Rachel is eating.

She ticks many of the anorexic boxes. From a high-achieving yet emotionally unavailable family, Rachel experienced trauma early when her father died of cancer when she was six. From being an assertive, playful child, she became quiet, anxious, a girl who teachers remarked was carrying the weight of the world on her shoulders.

As she grew into adolescence, these traits grew with her, developing in complexity. The smallest things disturbed her – animal cruelty on TV, war footage shown in history classes, funny looks from some of the other girls at the grammar school she attended in an affluent part of Cheshire.

Like her older sister, who took an internship at Merrill Lynch in London, Rachel showed academic aptitude and was considered a polymath. She was particularly strong in English, with a flair for creative writing.

But her pathology had sharpening claws too. She developed an over-reliance on systems, structure and order in her outside world. Changes to schedules or disruptions to plans would throw her. Control was essential. And as her body began to change shape, growing into puberty, so too did a desire to stay in control of that.

'It began with the faddy diets,' her mum Cynthia, a corporate lawyer, tells me later. 'The usual teenage preoccupations. Worrying about how she looked. What others would think.'

We're speaking outside the ward where Rachel remains. Earlier, Cynthia had been asked to leave. The official line was that Covid restrictions remained in place; unofficially, I was told by the charge nurse that Cynthia's presence was causing Rachel undue stress. Judging by Cynthia's headmistress voice, the fact that she has a pen and clipboard and insisted on my full name and credentials before talking to me, I get a sense of where this stress might be coming from.

'She was never heavy,' Cynthia says. 'None of us in the family have ever been *fat*.' She spits the word, the sound like bacon hitting a pan.

'Why do you think this eating disorder has emerged now?' I say.

'Isn't it obvious? It's delayed grief. I don't think she ever got over the death of her dad. And it's made her become so ... so self-absorbed.'

I tilt my head.

'First, she became vegetarian. Then vegan. Then intermittent fasting. Calorie counting. Totting up numbers. On the rare occasions we ate out, she'd only let us go to Wetherspoons, places where they have the calories written next to each meal. Even then she would order a green salad. A couple of years back, she started doing well. She had a year of food abstinence.'

'Food abstinence?'

Cynthia tuts. 'You should know about these things. It's the equivalent of the alcoholic getting a year sober. No disordered eating.'

'Ah.'

'She was even talking about going back and finishing her schooling. Maybe applying for university.'

'What happened?'

'Lockdown.'

I nod.

'Everything was in flux. I was working from home. My other daughter stayed in London. It was just us, Rachel and me. We seem to trigger one another. I can't explain it.'

But facing Cynthia's stare, I suspect I can.

She goes on to tell me that she can't cope with Rachel returning home, living in this bubble, pretending things are OK; every morning she's petrified she will walk in and find her daughter dead.

I ask, 'How do you feel now? With her being treated here?'

Cynthia makes a snorting sound. 'How would you feel if it were your child?'

'I'd feel lousy,' I say.

'There's your answer. But if it will keep her alive, what else is there?'

I tell her I don't know, and she rubs her eyes, darkening the lids with a slash of mascara.

Of all the mental illnesses, anorexia has the highest mortality rates. Although borne in the mind, it attacks the body, and malnourished patients can go into organ failure and die fast.

Back on the ward, I tap the door to Rachel's room and come in. Telling someone that they are to be detained and treated against their will isn't something I look forward to, but it is imperative that Rachel be equipped with the facts. This isn't punishment, it's to save her life.

Next to her bed, someone has left a cup of tea and two digestives.

'So can I go home now?' she says. 'Back to Mum?'

I shake my head. 'I want you to stay here and get well.'

'I am well. Weren't you listening to me earlier?'

She makes a knot of her hands. Her fingers are like stalagmites. The pale skin covering her face seems to stretch over the bones.

'Try to stay calm,' I tell her.

'What are you on about? What do I need to do to get out of here?'

My eyes fall to the two digestives. Rachel's do too, staring at the biscuits as if they are kryptonite.

After leaving the CAMHS job, I took three months out from mental health nursing to finish my second novel.

The floundering and dishonesty of the government during

the Covid period, the abuses of power, manipulation of trust and sheer solipsism were drip-feeding into the news – every week came revelations of VIP cronies paid millions to produce shoddy PPE, cake and booze being consumed while the Queen buried her husband, public figures caught with their trousers down and their hands in the cookie jar. Elsewhere, the awful case of Sarah Everard's murder at the hands of a serving police officer caused a swathe of anger and mistrust for those in control.

The world seemed a cruel place. That second book reflected the tone, and it was a hard graft to finish. For the duration I live off the publishing advance, giving interviews about my well-received debut, having back-and-forth Zoom calls with editors and publicists, book bloggers and readers. I'm nominated for awards, feature in the press, talk at events where the most common question is, 'How has your day job influenced your storytelling?' For the first time I'm able to legitimately call myself a working author, something many writers imagine is the dream.

But writing is a solitary pursuit. Hours and days spent in a room, staring at a screen, alone in your head. Sometimes the characters turned up to work and I was able to knock out 2,000 words of first-draft prose, but other times they stayed hidden in the crevices of my imagination. I'd find myself morose.

It dawned on me that without the breadth of human interactions mental health nursing gave me, my well would soon run dry. I began missing the strange, familiar chaos. I'd also burned through my advance like a chain smoker and needed an income. So I returned, doing agency work for a while, eventually signing up full time, where my job was to assess patients under the Mental Health Act.

This, I found, meant a learning curve. Unlike London, a dense city spliced into boroughs, the northwest is sprawling, with a huge geographical footprint. There's towns and villages, hamlets and nameless roads, and reams of farms, fields, country lanes, bogs and marshes. There are pockets of affluence and wealth but these are pitted against communities ground down by the decline in industry and tourism, now rife with county lines drug dealing, addiction and poverty. What someone might pay for a modest house in London would afford a whole street of terraces up here. The rasp of exhaust fumes and city pollution is swapped for manure and wet grass. It is, quite literally, a different world.

But mental ill health talks a universal language, and, although the accents are different, the stories I hear are familiar. Rachel's case presents me with my first real dilemma in this new post. Partly because the decision to section her got under my skin. But also because the severity of her illness chimed with another anorexic young woman who relapsed during Covid.

Nikki Grahame was a contestant on the seventh series of *Big Brother*. Loud, effervescent, saucy, she had no filter and her directness and puerility were impossible to forget.

I was shocked to learn of her death in 2021. In a subsequent documentary, her mum revealed how hard Nikki had found the Covid restrictions, which disrupted her routines and her ability to plan and control the things around her. She was supposed to go into yet another private mental health facility for treatment. Before she could make it, her body gave up. It seemed such a waste, and the parallels with Rachel screamed.

Sadly, stories like these aren't uncommon. Recent years have seen a sharp spike of admissions for eating disorders, prompting the Royal College of Psychiatrists to launch MEED guidelines (Medical Emergencies in Eating Disorders) for frontline staff around the administering of urgent, life-saving care for acute cases. Children and young people seem to be particularly affected by these disorders, with a staggering rise of 90 per cent in a five-year period up to 2021, in females and males.

Why?

Whole books have been written on the topic. It's easy to blame peer pressure and unrealistic body shapes on social media or the fat-ism promoted by the Katie Hopkinses of this world. Anorexia-promoting, or 'pro-ana', sites are clearly pernicious, for they glorify self-starvation and purging, edifying users with ingenious ways to maintain their illness and deceive professionals while blasting them with images of emaciated bodies to emulate.

I suspect the root causes of eating disorders are as varied and complex as the sufferers. One recurring theme seems to be that need for control. In a world that seems to be fragmenting, cruel and unpredictable, restricting what you eat, totting up the calories, seeing the results on the scales might provide the same deceptive hit that an alcoholic gets from a drink.

Research shows that the earlier support is provided, the better the outcomes. There are many who were seriously ill as teens now living with relatively healthy weights and obsession-free. But for those in whom the illness is entrenched, and who struggle into adulthood, the future can be uncertain. Along with the lasting damage they may inflict on their internal organs, their bones and joints through malnutrition, their teeth through harmful acid from daily vomiting, there are the permanent scars the eating disorder mindset can leave. I've heard some anorexics personify their illness as if it's alive, feeding them misinformation, telling them they're fat, no good, ugly. The only way to placate the voice is through restriction. It must be exhausting.

With Rachel, right now, refeeding is the only option. Trying to reason with her illness is like penetrating a battle cruiser with a knitting needle. But the traumatic impact intrusive feeding might have on her can't be downplayed. Imagine if that was your family member? What scars would be left long term?

As I leave the hospital, return home to Spencer and watch him chomp on his cheesy pasta with unbridled glee, it dawns on me how awful it must be to know your child is being held down and renourished through plastic tubes.

I next see Rachel three months on. By now, she's been transferred from the general hospital ward to a private mental health unit specialising in the treatment of eating disorders.

Specialist eating disorder units – SEDUs – are regimented places. They are governed by routines, surveillance, observation, negotiation, the staff trying to forge rapport while monitoring patients' dietary intake. These staff, for obvious reasons, will become preoccupied with numbers, evidence of weight loss and weight gain, meal plans and folders of spreadsheets, stats and charts. Nothing a patient says is taken for granted, and all their promises and assurances must be scrutinised against those cold hard digits on the weighing scales.

Walking around the grounds of this SEDU, the patients are easy to spot – thinness being a defining quality. But this is a certain type of thin: a defiant, wilful, angry kind. One young woman, walking with a chaperone, looks at me as I pass. Her eyes bulge like billiard balls. She is wooden in her baggy raincoat. Her mousy hair has patches missing and her skin is like chamois. She could be anywhere between fifteen and fifty.

I've come here to discuss Rachel's discharge from the unit and the proposal to place her on a community treatment order. CTOs are used for patients with established mental disorders who may need to be recalled swiftly, should they lapse. For some, being on a CTO is helpful, containing, for it provides a structure for them and their care team to adhere to; for others, it feels like being tagged, where you are never free and can have your freedom removed at a whim.

Rachel's inpatient doctor is adamant that a CTO is appropriate. To remain out, she must maintain a certain weight and allow health professionals to monitor her. On paper it seems reasonable, but I need to find out what Rachel has to say.

I'm shown into the office. A staff nurse hands me Rachel's notes. The file is fat, the information dry and impersonal, punctuated with units and percentiles, food and fluid intakes, bowel movements, blood levels.

A lot of it goes over my head, but the general gist is that

Rachel has responded well to support and treatment, and her ability to tolerate feeding and weight gain has improved. She had a rocky start, resisting feeding at every mealtime, requiring restraint and two-to-one monitoring. Eventually, she became more accepting, and attempts were made to remove the feeding tubes and give Rachel the agency of eating for herself.

'How's her mood been?' I ask one of the nurses, who stares at me strangely over the rim of her mug.

'Has she been responding well to support?'

'Rachel's Rachel,' she says. 'But her weight has improved. See?' She points at the weight charts before me.

I thank the nurse and tell her I'd like to see Rachel now.

Rachel is eating lunch.

She's in the dining room, the sole patient, sitting at a table in front of a plate of pasta. A staff nurse stands behind her like a sentry, surveying her. Rachel appears to be in a fugue. Eyes closed. Breathing diaphragmatically. At first I'm unsure what I'm seeing. Then it lands – she's praying.

A moment later her eyes reopen. She looks at the pasta the way a pathologist looks at a cadaver. Slowly, meticulously, she lifts her fork. She spears a pasta tube. She bites off the tip.

There is something private to this scene I'm witnessing, an effort of immense focus that shouldn't be disrupted. She continues eating in this manner, fork to mouth, one pasta tube after another, until the plate is empty. The process lasts ten to fifteen minutes. Finally, the nurse takes her plate and leaves, nodding at me on her way out.

SOME GIRLS ARE BIGGER THAN OTHERS

I enter the room.

Rachel has put on weight. It's in her cheeks, her neck, her hands and wrists, every part of her nourished and reinflated. By no means heavy, her body, dressed in khaki chinos and a lilac shirt, has shape. There's meatiness around those jutting shoulders, a slight swell to her chest and rear. There's colour to her skin too, and her hair looks thicker, richer.

'Great to see you again,' I say, and take a seat. 'How've you been getting on?'

'Fine,' she says, looking at the table. The tangy pear-drop smell of ketosis has gone from her breath. 'I've been working hard on meal plans. Engaging with the dietician. Focusing on the future.' Her words are genuine, but the delivery is listless, like she's reading from an autocue.

'That's why I'm here,' I say. 'To talk about the future.'

'I want to come out.'

'How do you think you'll cope?'

'I'll have Mum.'

'Do you think you'll be able to eat?'

'Of course. Weren't you listening?' She looks up. I can see it then – a hungry sickness in her, wailing to be heard.

'I am listening,' I say.

There is a silence. And she talks.

About her fears of staying in hospital, and her fears of going home with her mum and reverting to how she was. She tells me about her fear of eating, of not eating, of being honest with people, of lying to them. She tells me how she wants to get better, but she wants to be ill too, and the tug of war is exhausting. Her body might be thriving, but she misses that sense of control she had.

'I know I'm better right now.' She looks down at her body, at her full belly. 'But I feel so disgusting.'

'You're not disgusting,' I say, aware a comment like this will fall on deaf ears.

She nods. 'All the doctors and nurses here say the same. But when I look at myself in the mirror . . .' she clamps an inch of non-existent fat on her tummy between thumb and forefinger, 'I hate it. Like I'm the ugliest person on the planet.'

It's demoralising to hear this bright young woman talking about herself in this way. This is a vulnerable time for Rachel: she's approaching a healthy weight. But she still has the mind of an anorexic. It will take a lot of work to build up a counter-defence.

'What do you want to do with your life?' I say.

'I want to go to university,' she says. 'And study English. Maybe write one day.' She pauses. 'Like you.'

'Me?'

'Mum googled you. You wrote a book, right?'

My cheeks heat up. She looks back at the table where her plate had been.

'What do you think should happen next?' I ask. 'To help keep you well?'

'I don't know,' she says.

'Do you want to stay here at the hospital?'

'No.'

'Do you want to go home?'

'No.'

'Do you believe you can stay well and head off to university and win the Booker Prize?'

She begins to cry.

That afternoon, I sign the Community Treatment Order papers, and the following morning Rachel is discharged from the eating disorder unit subject to powers of recall, should her anorexia relapse.

Cynthia, her mum, takes this news as a personal insult. 'Ridiculous! You don't think I can keep my daughter well?'

'It's in no way a reflection of your parenting,' I say. 'It's an additional safeguard. She's been so poorly recently. And she's not out of the woods yet.'

'Well, if you ask me, it's a breach of her rights. I'll be complaining.'

I give her details of who to complain to and she scratches down the information using her clipboard, her eyes fizzing with reproach.

The prognosis for patients with treatment-resistant anorexia is mixed. The National Institute of Clinical Excellence (NICE) acknowledges that recovery rates dip the longer the person has the illness: estimates suggest that 46 per cent of people recover fully, 34 per cent improve partially, and 20 per cent develop chronic anorexia from which they never fully emerge. Early intervention is important, for the outcomes are demonstratively better in young people with a short illness duration – up to 60 per cent of adolescents with anorexia make a full recovery when provided with specialist treatment. But the relapse rates are high, and mortality rates are over five times greater in anorexics than in the general population.

Occasionally, services are forced to concede that all available options have been exhausted, and to continue with invasive procedures would be disproportionate and fruitless.

A recent case came to media attention that exemplifies such a controversial situation. BG, a nineteen-year-old anorexia patient, was allowed to have her support removed. A court hearing ruled that all options had been exhausted and further treatment was inflicting more harm than good.

For years, BG had been subject to refeeding, psychological therapy, assertive efforts to save her from starvation and dehydration, but to little avail. Upon discharge from hospital the illness would relapse, her weight would drop and she and her family would be forced to relive the hamster wheel of recall to hospital and refeeding again.

The judge concluded that she lacked capacity to understand the impact her anorexia was putting upon her, but that her wish to die through lack of food and water, endorsed by her exhausted parents and the professionals who knew her, was, on balance, the appropriate course. BG was allowed to return to the family home and passed away two months after the ruling.

Was this the right thing to do? At the time there were some who insisted she should've been kept alive and that the state was complicit in the needless death of a vulnerable person. But others accepted that in acute and chronic cases, there comes a point where professionals must accept their limits.

Rachel's discharge home lasts a paltry three weeks, by which point she's dropped seven kilos and is refusing to be seen by professionals. Swiftly, she is returned back to the eating disorder unit. She offers explanations for her weight loss – a bout of gastric flu and toothache, meaning she couldn't tolerate solids – but it's clear she has been restricting.

The last time I see her is at the SEDU. Nurses are restraining her, inserting the nasal-gastric tubes to commence refeeding.

It seems brutal. But so is anorexia.

As she fights and struggles, her screams fill the hospital corridor, formless and guttural, as if torn loose from inside her.

I head towards the exit knowing those screams will haunt me long after I've gone. There is nothing else to say.

Stretch Out and Wait

'When you forget where you left the housekeys, it's irritating,' Gerald says, leaning back on the sofa, his green eyes twinkling. 'That happens to everyone, doesn't it?'

'Yes,' I say. 'Mine went down the back of the sofa the other day.'

'When you forget where your house is, well–'

'You know something's amiss,' Sue, Gerald's slight, avuncular wife adds, sitting next to him, clasping his large hand in both of hers.

Gerald laughs. A laugh coloured with confidence and charisma, paired with a youthful smile that belies his seventy-six years.

I smile back. Sue looks away.

Gerald has been telling me about the most recent time he lost his house. On this occasion, six days back, the retired hotelier had just done eighteen holes on the golf course, had a meal at the clubhouse, was feeling energised, purposeful, and was driving his vintage Rolls home, a route he'd been doing years. Then, without warning, he found himself 'foggy'. He ended up circling the same stretches of road, stopping, starting, becoming exasperated. Eventually, police pulled him over for driving erratically. They removed his driving licence and contacted Sue.

There have been other foggy incidents too – putting a stapler in the fridge; leaving the gas hob running; mistaking a neighbour for a schoolfriend who died in the 1990s – all symptoms of the illness Gerald had diagnosed last month after weeks of tests, and which I'm here to talk to him about.

We're in the couple's six-bedroom Victorian house, a grand, palatial property in the affluent pocket of east Lancashire where they've lived for forty years, raising three children, hosting myriad Christmases, birthdays, Sunday dinners, the quarry tiles and oak banisters cured with memories. Warm smells of baked scones fill the house, ready for when the grandchildren come over later. Two beagles, Monty and Reggie, sit in wicker baskets by the hearth.

By today's standards, seventy-six isn't old, and Gerald could pass for younger. He's wearing preppy chinos and a pressed Ralph Lauren polo, smells of pricey cologne and has oil brushed through his iron-grey hair. There's a light dusting of crows' feet around the eyes, the slight shoulder stoop and hip stiffness when he stands, but he is ripe and healthy, brimming with interest. Yet in his head there exists a gremlin that isn't going away.

'Are you named after that actor?' he says to me.

'Which actor?'

'Elliot Gould?'

I tell him I'm not sure.

'We like his films, don't we, love?'

Sue nods.

'We've been watching old films from our courting days, then reminiscing about them. The doctor said keeping the mind active like that can help delay the changes.'

'Yes.'

'But the changes can't be stopped,' Sue adds.

'Correct.'

'Dementia,' Gerald says. 'In a sense, it's helpful to clarify why I'm getting like this. But knowing this thing's in me, well, it's changed my outlook. Made me realise that things will decline. At some point, I'll be a burden.' He looks at Sue. 'Then it will be time to take control.'

Something passes between them, an intuition with couples who've been together a long time. The kind of mental connection only years of companionship brings. Telepathy.

Gerald's GP asked me to attend today. A day prior, Gerald went to an appointment, collected his prescription for Donepezil, designed to ease dementia symptoms and delay the degeneration caused by the illness. When the GP asked how he was in himself, Gerald let slip that he was not planning to let his illness run its natural course. He would do everything he could to slow the decline, taking pills, keeping his brain active, exercising; he'd live life to the full, travel with Sue, tick as many things as he could off the bucket list. But when the time was right, he would take control.

Control.

Understandably, the GP took this to mean that Gerald was planning to end his life. On cue, he made a referral to mental health services, wanting us to assess whether he needed to be in hospital to stop him. Enter me.

'So how will you know,' I ask, gently, 'when it's time to take control?'

Sue winces.

'Well, it won't be for a while,' Gerald says, detaching his hand from hers. 'There's life in this old boy. We're flying to Canada next month. And come rain or shine, I'm determined to go up in a hot-air balloon. You ever done that?'

I shake my head.

'But when a man can't brush his teeth or attend to his toileting, it's time to have a serious look at what's for the best, don't you think?'

Sue winces again. 'I can take care of you, love.'

'But I don't want you to,' Gerald says, finding her eyes. 'I want us to have our time together in happiness, and then for you to enjoy however long you have without worrying about me.' He gestures towards the dogs. 'You wouldn't keep those two alive if they were in pain, would you?' He looks back at me. 'No, I've made up my mind. I've seen what this illness does to people. It's not for me. Thank you for visiting and showing an interest. You seem a conscientious young man, but I'll ask you to let me be. My decision is made.'

There's no point trying to argue. Gerald isn't going to budge. He's a man who has held boardrooms captive, managed teams, overseen vast budgets and projects, instigated lasting change; he's a successful businessman, a handicap-seven golfer, a former Scout leader, PTA chair, half-marathon runner; he's a pragmatist, unversed in the milky frailties that are segueing into his life but which will lead to him losing the essence of who he is.

'So what will you do,' I say, 'when the time's right? Go to Dignitas in Switzerland? Or have you planned something here?'

Gerald taps his nose. 'Mum's the word, I'm afraid. Suffice to say, I've prepared.'

'Prepared?' A cool draft seems to cut through the warm baking aroma in the house.

'There are people who give advice. I wouldn't want to jeopardise their trust, but I know what's needed.'

Sue doesn't wince this time. She is silent, but her eyes have a haunted look.

'And there we have it,' Gerald says, breaking the stiltedness with a chuckle. 'Did Sue offer you a scone?'

In *The Man Who Mistook His Wife for a Hat*, renowned neurologist, memoirist and all-round nice guy Dr Oliver Sacks remarked: 'A life without memory is no life at all.'

I can't imagine living without memory. Can you? Not knowing who, why or how I've come to be where I am – it seems inexplicable. Yet as the wonders of medical science increase life expectancy, diagnoses like Gerald's, predominantly associated with ageing, are becoming increasingly common. Everyone knows someone with age-related memory problems. Despite breakthroughs in the identification and prevention of dementia, at present there is no known cure for this cruel, terminal illness.

The adage Gerald used is one I've heard: if a pet gets ill, and it isn't getting better, you take it to the vet to be put down. Faced with a terminus as certain as dementia, why wouldn't you make plans to choose your death while you still could?

There are different kinds of dementia, and its assault will vary from person to person. Some are aggressive and attack the mind incessantly; others are slow burners and the decline is subtle, like a woodpecker on a tree; some experience a loss of retrograde information, memories from the long ago past that have shaped us inherently; others suffer anterograde decay, a loss in recent and new cognitions about what we're doing, why we've opened the fridge, where we've left our slippers; and some experience a carpet bomb of degeneration, feeling their mind fragment, the fabric and texture of who they are unravelling into a heap of twine.

Old age mental health care, with its intrinsic links to social care, has taken a pounding in the years of austerity and cuts. The previous government would claim that Covid was the cause for the staggering resource deficits, but it's clear the fault-lines were there years before – the pandemic put a magnifying glass to it.

Gerald isn't as stricken as some of the dementia patients I see in A&Es, impoverished, alone and afraid. He has money. He has Sue. He has options. But these options are tainted by an awareness of what lies ahead. In that sense, dementia is an equaliser. It cares not for wealth or status. It is inevitable, complete. Dementia is.

My job is to determine whether there is a role for a mental health intervention with Gerald and his plan to end his life. This is as much an existential quandary as a social or clinical one.

On one hand, I want to uphold his right to privacy and agency. In his position, I too might be making plans to check out how and when I want to. But there are other factors to consider. Is he making a sound decision? Is anyone with vexatious interests applying pressure to access his estate? What if his attempt to end things went horribly wrong?

This subject of suicide and assisted dying is opaque in the UK. As I type, government votes have supported an assisted dying bill to go through to the next phase of consultation, but this legislation, if endorsed, would apply only to those with six months or less to live, and who have the mental capacity to make this decision. Dementia patients can go on for years, and as the mind degenerates, so too can that capacity to make crucial life and death choices.

Presently, if someone with an illness like Gerald's is committed to dying, they must either fork out large sums and make the arduous trip to places like Dignitas in Switzerland, or they figure out a plan in a DIY manner and do it themselves. Despite risks of prosecution, there are those who are compelled to assist people on this journey. They are often retired or practising health professionals with strong views on the subject. They know death is something we only have one go at, and they want to help people get it done right.

Organisations like Dignity in Dying and Friends at the End campaign tirelessly for reforms and compel us to keep up with the changes introduced in neighbouring countries. In Germany, for example, 'suicide-pods' have been rolled out, where the person can lie back in a space-age contraption, press a button, inhale the fumes and slip away. It sounds clean and effortless, but the opposition to these measures remains strong: some argue there is scope for abuse and that the risk of mistakes outweighs the benefits; others take a puritanical view, see life as sacred, and disagree with it being ended intentionally, no matter the circumstances.

By now, I've been in the game long enough to have an affinity with death. With every patient the subject is broached. Are you having thoughts of ending your life? Have you made plans? What protective factors stop you from following through? What gives you hope and pleasure?

It also boils down to capacity. Is Gerald's plan to end his life a capacious decision we should respect? Or has his dementia impacted on his functioning, the ability to weigh up pros and cons of a decision, impeding his ability to make sound choices?

After mulling it over, taking advice from several colleagues, asking a psychiatrist to meet Gerald and having a long talk with Sue, I conclude that nothing Gerald said suggested he lacked capacity about his plans. On the contrary, he is lucid, clear and compelling in his rationale for wanting to not be a burden when he becomes too infirm, despite Sue disagreeing. In other words, Gerald may be making an unwise decision, but this is something he is free to do, as are all of us.

I phone the GP, explain that although I appreciate his dilemma, I didn't deem it proportionate to intervene into Gerald's life.

'So you're doing nothing?' he says, exasperation pinching his voice.

'Well,' I say, 'sometimes doing nothing is the best thing to do.'

'What about these threats to top himself? Isn't that a concern?'

'Yes, but he's not divulged details about when or how he will do it. There's nothing illegal that's been disclosed.'

'So what should *I* do?'

'Respect Gerald's wishes,' I suggest.

There's a loaded pause. 'But I just feel for poor Sue. The impact this will have on her. She wants to care for him, but he won't let her. He's so proud. It isn't fair.'

'Maybe you can persuade him to see differently?'

'You've met Gerald. He's belligerent. I doubt it.'

I agree. 'Well,' I say, 'I'm sorry. If you need us again, you know where we are.'

Our call ends amicably, and, as I put the phone down, there is the flicker of doubt and it dawns on me that this will not be the last time I meet Gerald.

My premonition proves true.

It's six months later, during a particularly bleak night of lashing Lancastrian rain. Clouds mask the sky. The moon is hidden. I've been asked to go and assess an elderly male who's been taken to an emergency department in a confused, agitated state. When I see Gerald's name on the referral papers, the pieces start slotting together.

Emergency departments in the northwest are no laughing matter. These places are bursting at the seams, the waiting rooms piled high with the sick and infirm, children, adults, grannies, granddads, drunks, addicts. They stand, sit, slump, lie supine. There are screaming babies. Howling grown-ups. The smell of vomit, urine, sweat, bleach and desperation scourges the warm, claggy air.

From behind a thick glass partition a receptionist does her best to help, guiding patients to toilets and vending machines, reassuring each that they will be seen, but the current wait time for non-emergencies is ten hours. Ten hours. And that's just to get triaged.

When it's my turn, I flash my ID. Fast, against the baying glares of patients, the receptionist ushers me through into the intestines of the A&E department.

It feels like I'm stepping into a warzone. I navigate around stretchers and wheelchairs, for every available public space is taken up with a sick patient. Some have wounded limbs or hold bandages to heads; some cup sick bowls and have drips feeding into veins. Most are elderly. Men and women who've worked hard, paid into the system and assumed that system would care for them. Now they endure pain in public, for the NHS is on its knees, with not enough room or staff.

A gaunt old man, clearly psychotic, is laughing hysterically as he sits on his stretcher, a blanket wrapped around him like a toga. A younger man, doubly incontinent judging by the miasma wafting from him, stares glumly ahead. A third, brittle old woman lies limp on a stretcher, eyes closed, lips parted. She could be asleep. She could be dead.

Nurses and doctors, paramedics and health care assistants all scurry from patient to patient, checking heart rates, taking blood pressures, administering pain relief, doing their best. But this isn't the kind of health care they were trained for. This is firefighting.

Amid it all is Gerald. Somewhere.

'Have you checked bay seventeen?' a forlorn charge nurse

says when I ask for help finding him. 'That's where he was last time I checked.'

I tell her I have checked bay seventeen, and bay sixteen, and eighteen, and he wasn't in any of them. She punches his name into a keyboard.

'Looks like they moved him again to free up space,' she eventually says. 'He was trying to leave. Doctor wrote him up for some benzos. They've got him in the prayer room.'

'The prayer room?' I say, sure I've misheard.

She shakes her head, sighs. 'Follow me.'

While we're pushing through the tide, she fills me in on what she knows. Earlier, Gerald had been reported missing by his wife. A few hours later, he was found by police wandering through the rain, wearing slippers and a flimsy shirt, soaking and confused. After some to-ing and fro-ing, they made the decision to bring him to A&E.

'We get a lot of these,' the charge nurse says, walking ahead, oblivious to the cries from the stretchers on both sides of her.

'A lot of what?'

'Old folk, losing their marbles, getting dumped on us. Family don't know what to do. Police don't know what to do. Social services don't know what to do. So they bring them here, thinking we have a magic wand. But this is A&E, not a bleedin' old people's home. We've got no space left.'

This charge nurse – Jade, according to her lanyard badge – lives up to her name, for she is jaded, ground down, fed up. I want to put her right, tell her she should be proud of what she does, that everyone deserves to be cared for ...

But I bite my tongue. Jade, no more than twenty-five, is working in the eye of the storm. This isn't the type of nursing she trained for. This is rearranging furniture on the *Titanic*. Behind her false eyelashes and filled lips, she's exhausted.

The prayer room is a cramped space meant for multifaith worship, not holding patients. Presently, Gerald is seated in a plastic chair, bare-chested, with a lime-green blanket around his shoulders. His iron hair is now a mop of grey scraggles, his purposeful stare a vegetable broth. The essence of him seems to have diluted, replaced with uncertainty, discord, dis-ease.

A cup of tea sits by his feet, along with a pill tub containing his next dose of temazepam, a sedative. Two security guards clad in high-vis vests and with crackling walkie-talkies stand at either side of him.

'Why's he with Security?' I say.

'He got a bit unhappy when we tried getting his wet clothes off,' Jade whispers, then looks at Gerald, enunciates loudly: 'We had to help you get changed, right, love? You'd have caught your death otherwise.'

'You don't need to shout,' Gerald says. 'I'm not deaf.' He looks at me.

'Hello again,' I say. 'Do you remember me?'

Gerald shakes his head.

I tell him my name, flash my ID. 'We met at your house. It was a few months back. I came over to see you and Sue.'

'The gardener?'

'I'm a nurse.'

'A nurse?' He chews on the word.

'Have you been feeling a bit foggy again?'

'Who are you? I don't believe you're a nurse.'

'Where are you now, Gerald? What is this place?'

He looks at the two security guards, Jade, and back at me. 'Is it a hospital?'

'Correct. Can you remember how you got here?'

'The police. They forced me. Put me in handcuffs. Then these two apes appeared from nowhere and dragged me and–'

The door opens, and we all turn. A woman with a Bible and a harried stare looks at us, says, 'Isn't this the prayer room?'

'Won't be long, love,' Nurse Jade says.

'But I want to–'

'I said we won't be long!'

The woman tuts and goes.

I return to Gerald. 'Where's Sue? Does she know you're here?'

A bereaved look falls across Gerald's face. 'Sue,' he says.

I wait.

'She was upset. We were both upset.'

'Yes?'

'I did something. To upset her.'

A cold tap drips inside me, putting me on edge. I'm about to ask more, but a fraught voice from outside the room beats me to it. 'Where is he? I need to know he's OK!'

In storms Sue, eyes wide, face frazzled. She looks old, thin, tired. A mousing bruise purples the skin on her left cheek.

'Thank God,' she says, and comes to Gerald, wrapping her arms around his neck. Gerald pulls his head away, like a schoolboy swerving his mum's affection in public.

'Why's he here?' she says. 'I reported him missing so that he could be brought home. Not treated like a criminal.'

'We're here for his protection,' one of the security guards says. 'He's been a bit . . .'

'Unsettled,' the other says.

'Nonsense,' Gerald says. 'Utter poppycock.'

'What happened, Sue?' I say. 'Will you tell me?' Outside the room, there's the crash of stretchers, the beeps of machines, the howls of patients.

'His pills,' she says. 'He–'

'Stop it!' Gerald snaps, and then pushes himself up to a stand. 'This is nothing to do with these people.'

'Calm down,' Jade says, and gestures at the guards to intervene. The guards, a hand on each of Gerald's shoulders, push him back down.

'Get off me!' he says. They ignore him. Sue covers her mouth.

I stand in front of Gerald and usher her outside. The door closes, and Gerald's protests are masked by the cacophony from the rest of the hospital. Sue is shaking like a leaf.

'Talk to me,' I say. 'What's been going on?'

'Things have become worse,' she says conspicuously, as fresh tears roll down her cheeks. 'It's happened quicker than I thought it would. His memory. His stress levels. Sometimes he's still my Gerald. Other times, he gets angry. Lashes out . . .'

I point to the bruise. She touches the skin, nods and whispers, 'This morning, he decided that it was time to take his pills.'

'Pills?'

'For ending things. He had them hidden, ready.'

I nod.

Her face scrunches up. 'But then he couldn't remember where they were.'

'Jesus,' I say under my breath.

'And when he couldn't find them, he blamed me.'

It's more tragic than I thought: the dementia patient who forgot where he stashed his suicide pills. I suspect Gerald, a perspicacious man, would've laughed at the irony. Once. Now things are too far gone. Put simply, he's left it too late.

'What happens now?' Sue says.

Good question.

Later, Gerald gets turfed from the prayer room and moved back to a corridor of the A&E department. He assures staff he won't try to leave. The security guards go on their break.

Gerald lasts ten minutes, but the noise, the distractions and the sedatives given earlier wearing off prove too much. Before long he's on his feet, shooing off staff nurses and Sue, trying to leave. Security gets called back. There's howling before more sedatives are given. He's held down on the stretcher until the meds kick in. Eventually, he dozes off.

By this point, I've already called two psychiatrists with the plan of assessing Gerald and getting him admitted to an older adults' mental health ward. I expect Sue to be all for an admission now, given how volatile the situation has become. To my surprise, she's ambivalent:

'I've seen people go into hospital and never come out,' she

says. 'It happened to my mum. I don't want that for Gerald. I want him with me.'

'But it isn't working at the moment,' I say. 'Is it?'

She shakes her head, looks at Gerald, snoring.

'I don't think it's safe for Gerald to come home,' I say. 'He could hurt you. He could hurt himself.'

'That won't happen.' She tries to inject some incredulity into her voice, but I see the puce of doubt in her eyes.

When the two psychiatrists arrive at the hospital a short while later, we have a debrief and talk about Gerald's diagnosis. Both are experts in older adult psychiatry. They know the score better than me.

We carefully rouse Gerald and speak to him in another poky room. At first, he puts on the charm, but it doesn't take long for the faults to show, cracks in memory, confusion, agitation. When the possibility of a mental health hospital is suggested as an option, he becomes infuriated.

'You can't be serious?'

'It would just be for a short while,' I say.

'But I'm not crazy.'

'I know.'

'So why do you want to send me to a madhouse?'

'I want you to be safe.'

'I *am* safe. Let me go home. Let me have control. *Please.*'

There's a pleading tone to his voice, laced with supplication, but his eyes are lit with rage.

Sue's concerns that Gerald would get worse in hospital are understandable. Removing anyone from their community and placing them in a mental health ward will be a shock to the system. But for a retiree in his seventies with an aggressive dementia, as Gerald's clearly is, it can be disorientating and lead to a rapid decline. If it were my parent, I'd hate it.

Recent public health research has shown that older adults with dementias are at higher risk of death in hospital during long stays – also in subsequent care homes – and immediate risks while admitted such as delirium, falls, dehydration, malnutrition, decline in physical and cognitive function and acquiring new infections. I've seen elderly people go into hospital opinionated and rambunctious and, after a matter of weeks, become feeble and vague, declining fast. Therefore, to proceed with an admission should be a considered, collective decision where benefits are balanced against risks.

The two psychiatrists and I discuss next steps with Sue. One consideration is to attempt a less restrictive option – send Gerald home and put in support from the home-treatment team. But that team are woefully short-staffed and cannot see him for three days; even if this could be expedited, I'm not convinced that a nurse doing a home visit for an hour would be enough to keep Gerald, or Sue, safe. An alternative is a respite facility, available for short-stay placements, but these are few and far between and, given Gerald's current volatility, I doubt many would accept him. The only other option is to section him.

'Will the hospital you send him to be near to home?' Sue asks. 'I want to be able to visit. Bring the dogs.'

'I don't know,' I say.

She looks at the floor.

We agree that hospital is the only choice we have.

As the two psychiatrists write their recommendations for this, we start making calls to see if there are any appropriate beds. Sue goes back to Gerald, dozing in a bay. When she takes his hand, his eyes flicker open. They share that look again.

It is predicated by the Royal College of Psychiatrists that by 2035 the number of people aged eighty-five and over will be approximately two-and-a-half times more than the figure in 2010, and the population aged sixty-five and over will account for 23 per cent.

Despite these data, the stock of old age mental health beds in the UK has dropped, with a greater drive towards crisis reduction and contingency planning in the community as alternatives to admission. The government argue that fewer admissions is a good thing, for it empowers patients, is less restrictive and reduces the risks of dependency and contagion.

But another uncomfortable truth is that slashing hospital beds saves money.

When I ask if there is a bed Gerald can be admitted to, the patient-flow manager sighs heavily down the phone. 'Call back in an hour,' he says.

I call back. Nothing.

Meanwhile, Gerald and Sue share a fractured sleep, him supine on the stretcher, her beside him on a fold-up chair. Day staff hand over to night staff. Charge nurse Jade scoots off; someone else takes over, equally weathered. A patient is rushed to resus. A bloody-nosed man is brought in by police. From the smell and commotion, the incontinent patient has had another accident. Outside, the rain keeps raining.

STRETCH OUT AND WAIT

At a quarter to midnight, there's a result.

'I've found somewhere that'll accept him,' the patient-flow manager says, 'but it's a bit of a way out.'

'How far?' I say through a yawn.

'County Durham.'

I check Google Maps. It's over a hundred miles away, a different part of the country. I look at an exhausted Sue, stiff and cold, next to a snoring Gerald.

Gently, I tell her the news. She bursts into tears.

'No,' she says, dabbing her eyes. 'That's too far.'

I agree. Inherently, it seems wrong for Gerald, who has never been admitted to a hospital, to be carted off to one that's hours away. But what are the alternatives? He can't stay here. And he can't go home.

'I'm sorry, Sue,' I say. 'Fingers crossed it will be temporary.'

'What if he gets worse?'

'He's going to a specialist unit. They know what they're doing.'

She plugs the name of the hospital into Google. A litany of 'requires improvements' CQC ratings blasts from the screen. Any remnants of hope fragment in my heart.

Sue looks up.

I try to smile, but it's as see-through as I feel.

A short while later, Gerald is roused by a staff nurse, given a cup of tea, a digestive and another dose of temazepam for the journey, and asked if he needs to open his bowels. Meanwhile, an ambulance crew appears – three burly men, their vehicle outside.

'Who are they here for?' Gerald says.

'They're going to take you to the hospital,' I say. 'We talked about it. Remember?'

He doesn't. Right now, I don't think he remembers who I am, or what's going on.

'I don't need to go to hospital, thank you very much. Sue? Sue! Take me home please. Now.'

Sue is already in tears. 'It's for the best, love,' she says through sobs.

'No,' Gerald says, the astute man he once was shining through the fog. 'I will not go.'

I look at the ambulance crew. They step in.

Restraint is a tough but necessary part of the job. Sometimes, there really is no choice but to get 'hands-on'. On paper, I understand the grounds for it, but man, is it grim to see.

Gerald isn't going without a fight. Despite the sedatives, his age, his apparent frailty, it takes the crew on each arm, plus two new security guards, a staff nurse and me to hold him down in a wheelchair and convey him safely through the halls to the vehicle outside. He lashes and spits with the desperation of a drowning man, hurling abuse. People stare, laugh, grimace. A teenage boy starts videoing on his phone. Behind us, Sue is weeping.

The ambulance has a celled rear chamber. In the lashing downpour, Gerald is strapped into a chair, secure and immobile. Rain trickles off his brow. He shivers and cries.

'No! No!'

The doors slam and he stares out through the barred hatch.

'Will he hate me?' Sue says beside me, watching the

ambulance pull away. She is as still and unyielding as a deckchair.

I tell her of course he won't. For I'm hoping the obvious: tomorrow, Gerald won't remember any of it.

The next day, I call the hospital Gerald was admitted to, wanting to confirm he arrived safely and was doing OK.

After several attempts, an insouciant-sounding staff nurse picks up. At first, she isn't sure who Gerald is and puts me on hold while she goes looking. Flowery music fills my ears for five long minutes. Then she returns.

'Dementia patient brought in last night?'

'That's him.'

'Yeah, Ronald's fine.'

'His name's Gerald.'

'Sorry, Gerald.' I'm about to ask more, but she blurts, 'Hold on, pet, got an issue with a patient,' and goes.

The weeks pass, and Gerald fades from my memory. Other things take precedence. Enrolling Spencer into a reception class. Re-landscaping our back garden. Finding the best deals on car insurance. Grown-up stuff.

As Partygate dominates the headlines, and the sitting prime minister is made to squirm under the spotlight, it dawns on me that I'm no longer a young Londoner but a middle-aged suburbanite, settled down into a predictable lifestyle like Gerald and Sue no doubt were at my age.

My involvement with Gerald might've ended there. I'd done my job, tried my best with the resources available. But mental health work has a habit of surprising you, and a few months later, his name drops into my inbox again. The message is from the GP who made the initial referral. Once again, he's voicing concerns. I'm shocked to read that Gerald was discharged from hospital after only a week. Understandably, the GP is worried.

My first instinct is to be angry at the situation. Had that shoddy hospital discharged Gerald prematurely, without a robust care plan put into place?

When I arrive at their house, it looks as ostentatious as before – the Rolls in the drive, the hanging baskets fresh. But inside is another story. There's a tired, worn quality. The family photos have been removed, replaced with handrails, key-safes, alarms; arrows pinned to walls directing to the lounge, the loo, the stairlift. A commode sits in the hallway; judging by the smell, it's recently emptied and swirled with bleach; there are handprints on the walls, and two panes of stained glass have been boarded with card. The warm home I remember is now a clinical residence.

Sue forces a smile. Her skin looks porous and her eyes are wet and dirty.

'I've made some changes,' she says, 'since Gerald came out.' The bruise she had before has faded, but her hands are scratched, and age hangs on her body like a wet towel.

'I can see,' I say. 'I gather he was only in hospital a week?'
She nods.
'Why so brief?'
'I brought him home.'

I let this sink in. Sue exercised her rights as Gerald's nearest relative to request his discharge from hospital. The hospital, in turn, made no effort to keep him. Her devotion to keeping Gerald with her is commendable. And worrying.

'Wow,' I say. 'That's a lot of responsibility.'

'It was necessary. That hospital was killing him. I looked at a few care homes but they're the same. People decline fast in those places. Well, it won't happen. Not with Gerald.'

I study her. Despite the fatigue greying her, I know she means it.

'Let's take you through to say hello,' she says. 'You can see how well he's doing.'

I follow her into the lounge. Gerald is in an armchair, wearing a dressing gown over a tracksuit, watching TV, the sound turned down. There's a vacillating quality about him, there in his chewing jaw, his shaky hands, his vacant affect.

'It's good to see you again,' I say. Gerald looks up and offers his hand. His palm is cool and silky, but the grip still firm.

'And it's good to see you,' he says tremulously.

I sit. Sue perches on the sofa rest beside Gerald.

'How've you been?' I say.

'Fine,' Sue says. 'You're fine, aren't you, love?'

I stay with Gerald. His mouth keeps chewing.

'It's so much better here than at that dreadful hospital,' Sue says. 'We can go for walks to the high street, we can sit in the garden, we can be together. We're OK. Aren't we?'

Gerald grunts.

He doesn't understand. He doesn't know what we're talking about, who I am, or perhaps who Sue is. He's a rough sketch of the man he was. But there's still a remnant of him. And after perhaps a minute of static, the stylus drops, a twinkle comes back to those eyes, and I know he recognises me from somewhere distant.

'There are carers you can pay to assist you,' I say. 'Local agencies.'

'No thank you,' Sue says.

'At some point, things will become too much. You know that?'

'I'm fine.'

'What do you think, Gerald?' I say. 'Is there anything you want?'

'I . . .' he says and then falters.

'Are you happy living here? Just you and Sue?'

Gerald looks at Sue.

The air thickens between them.

Some would say that Sue is a hero; others, that she is mistreating Gerald, putting her needs ahead of his, and both their lives at risk. Some might say her refusal to accept help could be construed as a form of abuse, and there might be grounds to intervene. But I don't think we're there. I have concerns about Sue's ability to cope as a carer long term. She does it the way I'd probably do it – out of duty, out of love.

She's not alone. In a 2021 census, the estimated number of unpaid carers in the UK touched five million, around 9 per cent of the population. Of that, 59 per cent are women, and female carers are more likely to provide care for patients like Gerald, with complex needs. Between 2012 and 2020, 41 per cent of carers were at or approaching retirement age. Many have care needs themselves.

These are our silent soldiers. Without them, the system would collapse.

To prise Gerald and Sue apart would seem inherently wrong. So, as with my first visit, the outcome is to do nothing.

Before going, I give Sue some pamphlets on the Alzheimer's Society, Dementia UK, Carers Network, and urge her to contact them. She tells me she will, although I doubt she means it. That brief admission to hospital has soured her trust in services. She wants to be left alone.

'I can cope,' she says. 'Honestly.'

I call the GP, inform him that I'd visited and was impressed by Sue's dedication to Gerald and her commitment to keep him home with her.

'But they have money,' the GP says. 'Gerald could be in a care home.'

'But Sue doesn't want that.'

'It would make her life so much easier.'

'Perhaps.'

I suggest the GP refers Gerald to an older adults' mental health team so that a care coordinator and psychiatrist can review him regularly and check for any further decline. I encourage him to support Sue's physical and mental health, signpost her to carers' support networks, ensure her needs are being met. I share his concerns that their situation could quite easily implode.

'So what should I do?'

'Watch,' I suggest. 'And wait.'

A year or so later, while doing an audit of old case files, I look up Gerald's notes and see that he died a few months after that last visit. A major stroke. He was at home. With his dogs. And Sue. It's not the death he envisioned, but as deaths go, I'd like to think it was a good one.

Did we do right by him? It's hard to say. There's no rulebook for situations like these.

Getting old isn't easy. Now, entering my middling years, I can feel it too. That youthful sense of indestructability is gone. Life is tenuous. And precious. It's about communication and connection, choice and sacrifice, love and laughter. It's about that lasting look indelible on my memory between Gerald and Sue, and a palpable connection forging them.

Telepathy.

There is a Light That Never Goes Out

THERE'S SO MUCH more that could've been written in this book. Over the years, I've met colleagues who've said that they should write about all the experiences they've had on the job. Well, I'm lucky enough to have been given the chance to attempt that.

But an attempt it is. And I've had to settle with these stories, and hope they've given you that sense of the tribulations, grim and gratuitous, hilarious and harrowing, that come with being a mental health professional. To experience it properly, though, you'll need to jump in and try it for yourself.

In university we were introduced to the frameworks we were training for – the science, the standards, the codes and the practical skills we must adhere to in order to uphold our registrations. But this pithy education failed to teach us what being out there working with humans was really going to be like. How we could alter their futures for the better. And how doing so would alter us too.

This is a tough job. There are reasons to give up, slope away or not bother trying. There are the exorbitant student fees to do the training, the poor pay once you qualify, the maddening lack of resources, the fatigue, burnout, the risks to your own health and wellbeing the work brings.

Yet twenty years on I'm still here, as are many colleagues who've become friends. Why? What made us stay? I've asked various mental health professionals I know this very question. The answers, a selection of which are below, have been enlightening:

'Because I'd like the care I give to be the care I'd receive if I was ill.' – Hannah

'To help people. Simple.' – Attique

'Because there is nothing more important than relationships and connections.' – Jose

'There's nothing quite like seeing a patient in a psychotic state in seclusion get the right treatment and recover.' – Anthony

'I'm in it for the pension. End of.' – Anon

'Because patients deserve care and treatment that supports them to live a fulfilling life.' – Lianne

'Because I have a mortgage to pay.' – Jenny

THERE IS A LIGHT THAT NEVER GOES OUT

'Because it's important that people have someone who understands what living with mental health problems is like.' – JC

'Because there's no other job that surprises me like this one.' – Caroline

'Because it's a privilege.' – Mark

There you have it. This is an incredible job. And an awful one.

We see the best in people when the guardrails are lowered and the sap of raw emotion spills through. We see the worst too, the scars of cruelty, trauma, abuse, suffering and greed. There have been dark days when I've questioned what I'm doing – whether it is good for patients, for me, my family and what I value.

Yet when I've stepped back, I've missed it. For if you're interested in the emotions behind the look, the flicker in the saccharine smile, the tears behind the fake lashes, this is a vocation where you can search for answers.

I've collected a trove of memories. Not grand and theatrical; they are small, seemingly inconsequential, but real. Most recently, taking Spencer to his first football match at the Emirates, walking along Holloway Road amid the sea of red and white, spotting Jack's mum Mary. Alone. Clutching her bag of shopping.

For a fleeting moment our eyes meet. She recognises me, then sees Spencer, and we both know that her son Jack is gone. The unfairness of mental illness makes the football chants and traffic noises dull to the pinging of a tuning fork.

Then Spencer is pulling my hand, and the spell breaks. Mary goes her way. And I go mine, left only with hope for her. Hope is important. It was important in the football match we went on to see (we lost). And it's important if you're going to survive working in mental health.

I hope to survive another twenty years and not burn out or give up. I hope to see my son grow up in a society where mental health care is taken as seriously as other forms of health care. I hope someone reading this might consider working in mental health and find as much value and meaning as I have. I hope that stigma will be challenged, discrimination redressed, and that people accept that we're all as crazy as each other.

I hope.

Acknowledgements

Where to start?

Gordon Wise, for your perseverance and belief; Ciara Lloyd, for your positivity and reassurance; Flora, Eleanor, Saira, and all the team at Blink for your investment in and drive behind the project and subject matter. You guys rock.

There's fellow writers: Andrew Mettam, Bonnie Garmus, Lenny Henry, the late Amer Anwar, Jack Butler, Spread the Word, TLC, and the original CBC Tuesday night crew.

My family and friends: Jane, Jim, Aunt Sarah, Ol, Vicky, Alice, Sam, Charlie, Clare, Kia, Jose, and the big man, Spencer. I love you all.

Colleagues from the past two decades: Billy Campbell, Ollie Kemp, Alan G, Jo Malone, Nigel Yard, Allison Arekion, Mark Hammond, Karen Hacking, Jenny Hoyle, David Hamilton, Mary McGerr, Darren Jefferson, Erico Jacobi, Margaret Green, Dave Brooks, Steven Lockley,

Debbie Harding, Richard Mason, and pretty much everyone else I've had the good fortune to work with.

There's the mental health workforce – troopers fighting the good fight at this very moment; those who've devoted a career to supporting people in times of crisis and those considering or poised to enter the profession – you are welcome.

Lastly, there's the patients, past, present and in the future. Whoever you are, it is my privilege to know you.